Practising Social Work Ethics
Around the World

Ethics is an increasingly important theme in social work practice. Worldwide, social workers experience common ethical challenges (how to be fair, whether to break a rule, how to act in politically tense situations) in very different contexts – from disaster relief in China to child protection work in Palestine.

This book takes as its starting point real-life cases featuring ethical problems in the following areas: negotiating roles and boundaries; respecting rights; being fair; challenging and developing organisations; and working with policy and politics. Each case opens with a brief introduction, is followed by two commentaries and ends with questions for reflection. The commentaries, written by authors from different countries, refer to relevant theories, concepts, practical matters, alternative courses of action and their implications. Features within the book include:

- an introductory chapter covering issues of global ethics;
- cases and commentaries drawn from across the world – from Peru to Finland;
- cases based on real-life situations and chapter introductions from leading authorities in social work and ethical theory;
- questions and practical exercises to aid teaching and professional development.

This book is a unique and accessible resource for stimulating ethical reflection, expanding ethical horizons and developing ethical and intercultural sensitivity. It is designed for use by undergraduate and postgraduate students and professionals in the fields of social work, social education/pedagogy, social care work, international social work, community development, community organisation, youth work and related fields.

Sarah Banks is Professor in the School of Applied Social Sciences, Durham University, UK. She teaches and researches in community, youth and social work and is co-director of the Centre for Social Justice and Community Action. She is co-editor of the journal *Ethics and Social Welfare*, and author of several books on ethics for the social professions.

Kirsten Nøhr is a qualified social educator, MA in Higher Education, currently working at the Hogeschool van Amsterdam (University of Applied Sciences) in the Netherlands. She was a senior lecturer for social educators in Denmark for many years and co-editor of the journal *Dansk Pædagogisk Tidsskrift* (*Danish Journal of Education*).

Published in association with the journal
Ethics & Social Welfare

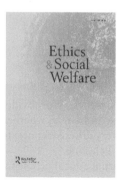

Ethics & Social Welfare publishes articles of a critical and reflective nature concerned with the ethical issues surrounding social welfare practice and policy. It has a particular focus on social work (including practice with individuals, families and small groups), social care, youth and community work and related professions.

The journal encourages dialogue and debate across social, intercultural and international boundaries on the serious ethical issues relating to professional interventions into social life. It contributes towards deepening understandings and furthering ethical practice in the field of social welfare. The journal welcomes a diverse range of contributions from academic and field practitioners, voluntary workers, service users, carers and people bringing the perspectives of oppressed groups.

Published By: Routledge
Frequency: 4 issues per year
Print ISSN: 1749-6535
Online ISSN: 1749-6543
www.tandf.co.uk/journals/esw

Practising Social Work Ethics Around the World

Cases and commentaries

**Edited by Sarah Banks
and Kirsten Nøhr**

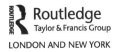

Routledge
Taylor & Francis Group

LONDON AND NEW YORK

First published 2012
by Routledge
2 Park Square, Milton Park, Abingdon, Oxon OX14 4RN

Simultaneously published in the USA and Canada
by Routledge
711 Third Avenue, New York, NY 10017

Routledge is an imprint of the Taylor & Francis Group, an informa business

British Library Cataloguing in Publication Data
A catalogue record for this book is available from the British Library

Library of Congress Cataloging-in-Publication Data
Practising social work ethics around the world : cases and commentaries
/ edited by Sarah Banks and Kirsten Nøhr.
p. ; cm.
1. Social service-Moral and ethical aspects-Case studies. 2. Social
workers-Professional ethics-Case studies. I. Banks, Sarah.
II. Nøhr, Kirsten.
[DNLM: 1. Social Work-ethics-Case Reports. 2. Internationality-Case
Reports. W 322]
HV10.5.P695 2011
174'.93613-dc22
2011003931

ISBN13: 978–0–415–56031–3 (hbk)
ISBN13: 978–0–415–56033–7 (pbk)
ISBN13: 978–0–203–80729–3 (ebk)

Typeset in Sabon
by Keystroke, Station Road, Codsall, Wolverhampton

Contents

Cases without commentaries

Using cases and commentaries in teaching and learning

List of cases by country

Tables

List of contributors of cases

Sonia Aguerri
Matthew J. Armstrong
Naimeh Baidoun
Peta-Anne Baker
Maryam Bibi
Erik Blennberger
Linda Briskman
Ana Bueno
Sema Buz
Adalberto Dias de Carvalho
Derek Clifford
Marilyn Crawshaw
Kiki Drion
Julie Drolet
Álvaro Faria
Melissa Floyd
Titti Fränkel
Leon Ginsberg
Allysa Gredling
Alison Higgs
Gloria Jacques
Jufitri Joha
Arja Jämsén
Grant Larson
Anne Liebing

Jane Lindsay
Igor Magalhães
Donna McAuliffe
Ashleigh Mercer
Marzieh Mirzaei
Marie-Geneviève Mounier
Rodreck Mupedziswa
Kerttu Ojalehto
María Jesús Úriz Pemán
Raquel Cuentas Ramirez
Miriam Samuel
Timothy Sim
Dalija Snieškienė
Frank Tesoriero
İpen İlknur Ünlü
Adele Valori
Abbas Ali Yazdani
Tan Yu
Aira Vanhala

Notes on editors and authors of chapter introductions

Sarah Banks is Professor in the School of Applied Social Sciences, Durham University, UK, where she teaches and researches in the fields of community, youth and social work and is co-director of the Centre for Social Justice and Community Action. She is co-editor of the journal *Ethics and Social Welfare*, and author of a number of books on professional ethics, including *Ethics and Values in Social Work* (Palgrave Macmillan, 2006), *Ethics, Accountability and Social Professions* (Palgrave Macmillan, 2004) and *Ethics in Professional Life: Virtues for Health and Social Care* (Palgrave Macmillan, 2009, with A. Gallagher).

Linda Briskman is Professor and holds the Haruhisa Handa Chair of Human Rights Education at Curtin University, Perth, Australia. She conducts research and publishes in the areas of indigenous issues and asylum seeker rights. Books include *Social Work with Indigenous Communities* (The Federation Press, 2007) and the co-authored *Human Rights Overboard: Seeking asylum in Australia* (Scribe Publications, 2008, with S. Latham and C. Goddard). Linda is a regular media commentator on asylum seeker issues, particularly detention on Christmas Island.

Derek Clifford is one of the founding co-editors of the journal *Ethics and Social Welfare*, and co-author with Beverley Burke of a book on *Anti-Oppressive Ethics in Social Work* (Palgrave, 2008). Now retired, he was formerly a Reader in Social Work at Liverpool John Moores University, UK.

Donna McAuliffe is an Associate Professor in the School of Human Services and Social Work, Griffith University, Queensland, Australia. She teaches and researches in the area of ethics and professional practice, and is the Convenor of the National Ethics Group of the Australian Association of Social Workers, leading the 2010 review of the Australian Social Work Code of Ethics. Dr McAuliffe has developed the inclusive model of ethical decision-making (with colleague Lesley Chenoweth), and has published a number of articles on ethical practice, ethical decision-making, and ethics in research.

Kirsten Nøhr is a social educator and MA in Higher Education, working as an educational consultant at Hogeschool van Amsterdam University of Applied Sciences, the Netherlands. She was a lecturer for social educators in Roskilde and Copenhagen, Denmark, for many years and a co-editor of the journal *Dansk Pædagogisk Tidsskrift* [*Danish Journal of Education*]. She has co-edited *Teaching Practical Ethics for the Social Professions* (FESET, 2003, with Sarah Banks) and *Etiske dilemmaer i pædagogisk arbejde* [*Ethical Dilemmas in Pedagogical Practice*] (Hans Reitzels Forlag, 2007, with Ruth Mach-Zagal).

María Jesús Úriz Pemán is Professor of Philosophy in the Social Work Department at the Public University of Navarre, Spain. She teaches and researches in the fields of professional ethics, epistemology, social work ethics and social philosophy. She has been the academic director of the Master in Social Welfare: Intervention with individuals, families and groups at the Public University of Navarre. She is Director of the research group EFIMEC (Ethics, Philosophy and Methodology of the Social Sciences). Dr Úriz is author of a number of books and articles on social philosophy, social ethics, confidentiality and autonomy in social work ethics.

Frank Philippart is a sociologist and lecturer at Avans University of Applied Sciences in Breda, the Netherlands. He teaches sociology, ethics and the methodology of social work. He has published on Socratic dialogue (including a chapter in *Teaching Practical Ethics for the Social Professions*, FESET, 2003) and gives training in Socratic dialogue. He is one of the founders of a national programme for the improvement of training programmes for forensic social work in higher education in the Netherlands.

Frederic Reamer is Professor in the School of Social Work, Rhode Island College, USA. His research, teaching and social work practice focus on criminal justice, public policy, and professional ethics. Recent books include *The Social Work Ethics Casebook* (NASW Press, 2009), *Ethical*

Standards in Social Work (NASW Press, 2010), *Social Work Values and Ethics* (Colombia University Press, 2006), and *Heinous Crime* (Colombia University Press, 2005). Reamer chaired the task force that wrote the current NASW Code of Ethics.

Foreword

Ethics is a subject of great importance for the social professions. I am delighted that FESET (Formation d'Educateurs Sociaux Européens/ European Social Educator Training) has been able to support the work that has gone into the publication of this book, which offers a unique contribution to the literature in this field. The book is the outcome of many years of work undertaken by the European Social Ethics Project, which is a working group of FESET with a focus on teaching, learning and research in the field of practical ethics for the social professions.

Hitherto the work of the European Social Ethics Project has been at a European level. In these times of increasing globalisation, and ever-growing challenges for social professionals working around the world, to have a book of international cases on ethics is of great value for practising professionals and for the education of students in the social welfare field.

Practising Social Work Ethics Around the World: Cases and commentaries 'fills the gap' as the theoretical and practical contributions in the book give the reader a good opportunity to reflect on social work in an international context, on the possibilities and problems related to the concept of 'global ethics', and also more generally on the relationship between universalism and particularity in ethics.

The value of the book is enhanced by very readable introductions to theories of ethics in social work and the social professions and by the way it introduces discussions about universal principles in local, cultural circumstances. The global nature of both the real-life cases and the commentaries will provide a valuable understanding of differences in social work practice, policy, law, culture and ethics in different countries and hopefully will strengthen the solidarity of social workers across the world.

The main aim of FESET is to promote education and training for socio-educational perspectives and to encourage collaboration between schools/universities that offer study programmes in social education at all levels – from professional Bachelors programmes, to Masters and Ph.D. level. This book constitutes an important contribution to these aims of exchanging ideas and issues and for finding common ground. Ethics is one of the fundamental aspects in practice, and for that reason the book will be an important analytical 'tool' for the preparation of students – including helping them in their reflections on practice, as well as in their cooperations with a range of professions in the social welfare field. This is particularly important for students undertaking international practice placements and studying international social work.

Inge Danielsen
President of FESET (Formation d'Educateurs Sociaux Européens/European Social Educator Training)

Preface

The main focus of this book, as its title implies, is a series of cases relevant to ethics in social work drawn from different countries, accompanied by short reflective commentaries written by practitioners and academics from around the world. The cases and commentaries are grouped into themed chapters (Chapters 2–6), each of which has an introduction written by an author with expertise related to the topic of the chapter. An introductory chapter (1) offers some background discussion on global ethics in social work and the nature of the cases. The final chapter (7) comprises some cases without commentaries for use in teaching and gives guidance on how cases and commentaries can be used in teaching and learning.

The book has a number of distinctive features, which we hope will make it useful for students, teachers and practitioners working in different countries and contexts.

- The cases are all taken from real life, and have been submitted by practitioners, academics and carers.
- The cases are drawn from across the world.
- The cases are written in a narrative format, and are longer and more discursive than typical short ethics cases.
- Some contextual details are given as background to each case – such as where it took place, and information about any relevant laws, policies, systems or norms.
- The commentators are drawn from across the world, with many offering their perspectives on situations with which they are unfamiliar.
- At the end of each case and its two commentaries, three questions for discussion are given, to stimulate reflection on the part of readers and groups of learners.
- The introduction to the book and the introductions to each chapter offer readers background theoretical and conceptual material, so the cases and commentaries are not left in a vacuum.

- A selection of exercises, tasks and guidelines is given in Chapter 7 as a guide to how to use the cases and commentaries in teaching and learning.

Origins of the book

The idea for this book was developed as part of the work of the European Social Ethics Project (ESEP) – a working group of Formation d'Educateurs Sociaux Européens/European Social Educator Training (FESET). Members of ESEP have worked together for many years (the group was formed in 1998), sharing ideas about the use of cases for ethics teaching and researching the ethical challenges faced by students. We developed a growing interest in 'ethics cases' – what counts as an 'ethics case', what makes a good ethics case and how cases can be used in teaching and practice development. Collaboration with colleagues from a variety of European countries also generated an interest in how students from different countries, cultures and backgrounds respond to the same cases. Some of this work was written up in a previous collection of materials from ESEP members, edited by Sarah Banks and Kirsten Nøhr (2003), *Teaching Practical Ethics for the Social Professions* (available free as a pdf file at www.feset.org/en/home/activities/thematic-groups/esep.html).

As Sarah became more involved internationally over the last few years, through the International Federation of Social Workers' (IFSW) permanent committee on ethics, and through attending IFSW and International Association of Schools of Social Work (IASSW) conferences, she felt it was time to move beyond Europe and consider some of the ethical challenges facing social workers in different parts of the world. Hence, she developed the proposal for this book and presented it to members of the ESEP group at its 10th anniversary meeting in Porto, Portugal, in 2008, when Kirsten Nøhr agreed to take on the role of co-editor.

Methodology for compiling the book

The plan of the book was based, from the start, around five predetermined themed chapters: negotiating roles and boundaries; respecting rights; being fair; challenging and developing organisations; and working with policy and politics. Each chapter would comprise four cases, with each case accompanied by two commentaries.

Cases were obtained by circulating calls for cases via professional associations and networks (European Association of Schools of Social

Work (EASSW), FESET, IASSW, International Federation of Social Workers (IFSW), Ethics and Social Welfare network), making announcements at conferences and directly approaching people at international conferences and meetings. Brief instructions were given on how to write a case and authors were requested to anonymise details of the case. The authors' identities would remain anonymous too, in order to safeguard the identities of service users and organisations.

Inevitably we received more cases than we could use in the book, and we had to make some very difficult choices about which to include. Our choices were constrained by our aim of having cases from a range of different countries, and needing cases on a range of different topics that would also fit with the chapter themes. A number of very interesting cases were not used in the book, but have been included on the website, www.feset.org/en/home/activities/thematic-groups/esep.html

By November 2009 we had received about 18 cases, which were reviewed by a small sub-group of ESEP at a meeting in York, UK. As we discussed which cases should be allocated to each chapter we could see that many of the cases could fit equally well in several chapters, as they had many ethical dimensions. We considered whether the existing chapter structure was helpful or not. Cases could have been grouped in other ways – for example, by service user group (work with older people, children or people with terminal illness) or by more specific topics (withholding information, child sexual abuse). In the end we decided to retain the existing chapter structure.

Although we had received 18 cases by November 2009 there were many more from Europe than elsewhere, and we were therefore unable to use them all in the book. We needed to make a concerted effort to obtain more cases from particular regions or continents. This was largely done through personal commissioning during 2010, particularly at international conferences. The last few cases were the most challenging – as we needed to fill gaps in particular chapters and draw in cases from countries not yet represented. The book became like a jigsaw puzzle. In the end, we were pleased with the spread of cases. With only 26 cases in the book, inevitably many countries are unrepresented. There are some parts of the world from which we did commission cases but which for various reasons did not arrive. We hope to remedy this on the website over the coming years.

For each case chosen for Chapters 2–6 there was usually a round of correspondence with the author(s) requesting more information, clarification and revisions. Our aim was to try to ensure that readers from many countries across the world would be able to grasp the main points of the case. Once the cases were revised we then sent them to commentators to offer a perspective on the case. Commentators were also given guidance (including in which chapter the case was to be located) and were chosen to reflect a range of different countries and expertise. When inviting commentators we relied on personal contacts, or knowledge of people's published work. None of the commentators saw the other commentary on the case they were discussing until the final stages of the compilation of the book, when each case with its two commentaries was sent to contributors for information and final checking.

Our original idea was that the chapter introductions should be written first, and might be sent to commentators as a backdrop against which to write their commentaries. The aim of the chapter introductions was to offer readers a concise overview of the topic of the chapter, not to discuss the cases in any detail (as commentators would do that). Some members of the ESEP group started to bring material together for these chapter introductions in 2009, but we then realised that it might make more sense for the chapter introductions to be written once most of the cases had been obtained. Most of the chapter introductions were finally written in 2010, and make brief references to some of the cases as illustrations, but do not discuss the commentaries. The commentators did not see the chapter introductions.

Our reflections

Working on this book has been both an extremely challenging and very rewarding experience. We have learnt so much about the conditions for and the practice of social work in many different contexts and countries and we are extremely grateful to all the contributors and our supporters for their willingness to engage in the project. We hope the cases and commentaries in the book will prove equally stimulating for readers, serving to inspire deeper ethical reflection and more concerted collective action in response to the many cases of injustice, abuse, courage and commitment experienced every day by citizens, service users, carers and social workers around the world.

Using the book

We hope we have compiled a versatile book that can be used in stand-alone sections. Particular cases can be read and discussed in their own right. A case with its two commentaries and three questions can also offer a stand-alone unit for study. Taking a chapter, with its introduction and four cases and commentaries gives scope for broader, theoretical and comparative discussions. Anyone interested in international social work and/or professional ethics in general might read Chapter 1 (which provides an overview) and any or all of the other chapters. Those who are teachers and want to use the book in teaching and learning contexts would be interested in Chapter 7, which offers suggestions for exercises.

Sarah Banks
Durham, UK

Kirsten Nøhr
Haarlem, the Netherlands

Acknowledgements

There are many sources of inspiration and support that have made this book possible. Although two names are on the cover as editors, the book is very much a collaborative venture.

As mentioned in the Preface, the idea for book was developed as part of the work of the European Social Ethics Project (ESEP) – a working group of FESET (Formation d'Educateurs Sociaux Européens/European Social Educator Training). Some members of the group have submitted cases that we have used in the book, others have written commentaries and yet others have contributed towards the introductory chapters. There are some whose names do not appear in the book as contributors, but who have contributed to thinking about the selection of cases to be used and the organisation of the book. We are particularly grateful to Victor van den Bersselaar, Maria do Rosário Serafim and François Gillet, for their participation in meetings in Porto, York and Osnabrück and also to Helene Jacobson Pettersson and Isabel Baptista for their continuing support and encouragement. Other members of the group who have participated in meetings and offered advice and support, as well as contributing cases, commentaries or chapter introductions include: Adalberto Carvalho, Anne Liebing, María Jesús Úriz Pemán, Frank Philippart, Dalija Snieškienė, Aira Vanhala and Agnes Verbruggen. We are also very grateful to the FESET board for financial support to help edit and collate cases not used in the book for the website. FESET has been a continuing source of support and a forum for the renewal of membership of the ESEP group since it was formed in 1998. The European Association of Schools of Social Work (EASSW), the International Federation of Social Workers (IFSW) and the International Association of Schools of Social Work (IASSW) also helped us in publicising our call for cases, as did colleagues on the editorial board of the journal *Ethics and Social Welfare*, and members of the Ethics and Social Welfare network.

We are very grateful to all those who contributed cases for this book. To preserve the anonymity and confidentiality of personal information relating to the service users, carers, professionals and organisations that feature in the cases, the authors of the cases are not attributed. However, these authors have put in a considerable amount of work in drafting and developing cases, often responding repeatedly to questions, comments and suggestions from the editors with great diligence and patience. Without their commitment, this book would not exist. We are particularly grateful to those who told their own stories with great honesty, and to those who made efforts to seek out practitioners in order to capture their stories and write them up. We are grateful also to all those who sent us cases which in the end we did not use. This was not because the cases were not interesting or challenging, but simply because we had to attempt to balance the numbers of contributions from different countries and wanted to ensure coverage of a range of different themes.

The commentators too deserve a deep debt of gratitude. We were delighted that people were willing to offer their perspectives on cases that were often far removed from their own expertise and experience, as well as on those cases that might be uncomfortably close. Again, these contributors showed great forbearance in responding to our suggestions for clarifying their commentaries.

The authors of the chapter introductions had a particularly difficult job. In most cases they drafted their introductions before seeing all the cases and certainly before reading any or all of the commentaries. They had a very difficult brief – to offer a concise introduction to the key ethical issues and concepts covered in each chapter. They rose to the occasion with alacrity and have set the scene for the chapters remarkably well.

We would like to acknowledge the particular inspiration drawn from the IFSW series of books, *Social Work Around the World*, and to thank both IFSW and IASSW for the wonderful opportunities provided by their conferences for meeting practitioners and academics from around the world and exchanging ideas and views. Recently, the conferences and meetings of the Social Work Action Network (SWAN) have provided a unique forum for developing solidarity and engaging in debate about the political context in which social work operates and the possibilities for holding onto concepts of radical social work with a genuine social justice purpose internationally. The work of Rona Woodward, Iain Ferguson, Michael Lavalette, Barry Levine and Mark Baldwin has been especially inspirational in this regard.

We would like to offer particular thanks to a number of people who have offered advice and support through discussions on professional ethics generally and in relation to particular aspects of the book, including:

Cynthia Bisman, Lena Dominelli, Ann Gallagher, Fumihito Ito, Michael Nieweg and Helle Strauss.

Finally, we must thank our editor at Routledge, Grace McInnes, who saw the value in the book and was willing to support the venture and to wait patiently for the delivery of the manuscript.

Global ethics for social work? A case-based approach

Sarah Banks

Introduction

This chapter provides an introduction to the book for readers who wish to reflect on the nature of social work in an international context and on the possibilities and problems of the concept of a 'global ethics'. A brief overview is given of a variety of theoretical approaches to ethics, followed by a discussion of the usefulness of case-based methods in exploring ethical issues internationally. A categorisation of the varieties of cases included in the book is given, including an analytical table at the end of the chapter.

It is not necessary to read this chapter in order to use the rest of the book. It may, however, be helpful for readers who are interested in considering the usefulness of ethical theories and in engaging in debates about universalism and relativism in ethics, and for teachers wishing to use the book with students.

Rationale for the book

Ethics in social work, and indeed in public life more generally, is a topic of growing importance. There has been a rapid growth in books and articles on this theme in the last decade (for an overview, see Banks 2008). There are many reasons for this so-called 'ethics boom'. The growing awareness of the impact of humans on the world environment and the potential for life changing bio-medical technologies are contributing to a heightened awareness of questions about the kind of world in which we want to live and the kinds of lives we should lead. The persistence of inequality, poverty and war, along with the phenomenon of global terrorism, the rise of neo-liberalism in politics, a retrenchment of traditionally strong welfare states, cutbacks in social services and a questioning of the expertise and trustworthiness of professionals bring ethical questions very much into the arena of social work. Social workers have to respond to asylum seekers fleeing zones of conflict, cuts in welfare budgets, privatising of welfare services and demands from employers that they act as gate-keepers, controllers or managers of care packages. The political and economic challenges confronting social workers vary across different parts of the world. However, there is no doubt that wherever in the world social workers practise, they face ethical challenges about how to treat and respond to people respectfully, how to ration resources fairly and whether and how to resist, ameliorate or tolerate the social injustices they see on a daily basis.

Despite the rapid growth of textbooks on social work ethics, there are relatively few that primarily comprise real-life social work ethics cases (Reamer 2009 and Rothman 2005 are examples from the USA) or that address the international dimensions of social work ethics in any detail. Specialist textbooks on social work ethics are more prevalent in the global North and West. Such textbooks usually cover ethical theories, codes of ethics and topics such as confidentiality, service user participation, rights and responsibilities, with case examples often used to illustrate different types of ethical dilemmas and problems (for example, Aadland 1998; Banks 2006; Beckett and Maynard 2005; Bowles et al. 2006; Charleton 2007; Congress et al. 2009; Dolgoff et al. 2009; Joseph and Fernandes 2006; Lingås 1992; Linzer 1999; Reamer 2006; Rouzel 1997). The aim of this book is to complement specialist texts on social work ethics, often written from a national perspective, and the growing number of books on international social work, which may have short sections or chapters on ethics (Cox and Pawar 2006; Healy 2001; Hugman 2010; Lyons et al. 2006).

Since discussion and analysis of accounts of practice in the form of cases is a well-used and very effective way of encouraging learning about ethical issues in social work, it is hoped that a book of real-life cases and commentaries will be a useful addition to the literature. The cases can be used in educational contexts to stimulate the development of skills in ethical perception and reflection and to generate dialogue about the roles, rights, responsibilities and dilemmas of professional practitioners, carers, service users, other professionals, politicians, social work agencies, governments and professional associations.

The inclusion of cases and commentaries authored by people from around the world has the added value of both enhancing understanding of differences in social work practice, policy, law, culture and ethics in different countries, whilst at the same time strengthening the solidarity of social workers across the globe. We hope the book will contribute to some of the important ongoing debates in social work about the extent to which ethical values are or should be shared internationally; and whether statements of ethical principles and standards can be valid universally, or whether they are always relative to particular contexts (Banks et al. 2008; Healy 2007; Hugman 2008).

Social work

We are using the term 'social work' in a broad sense to cover the work of a range of occupational groups operating in the social welfare field, including: social work; social care work; social pedagogy; social education; community work/community organising; and youth work. These occupations are configured differently in different countries, but broadly speaking they tend to work with individuals or groups of people who are judged to be in need of social services or social assistance; who may be thought to be a threat to themselves or others and therefore should be protected or controlled; or who may benefit from professional support, facilitation or informal education to take action themselves to work for individual and social change or transformation.

Even within the same country, there may be constantly shifting views of the purpose of social work, as economic, social and political conditions and regimes change over time. Payne (2000) offers a useful analysis, suggesting that the nature of social work emerges from a balance at any point in time between three shifting views of its purpose:

1　Maintaining the existing social order and providing individuals with services as part of a network of social agencies (*individualist-reformist views*).
2　Helping people attain personal fulfilment and power over their lives, so they feel competent to take part in social life (*reflexive-therapeutic views*).
3　Stimulating social change, transforming society by promoting cooperation, mutual support, emancipation and empowerment (*socialist-collectivist views*).

In many countries there are active professional associations of social workers, and in some countries there are state-sponsored regulatory bodies. These organisations publish documents outlining the nature of social work, the responsibilities of social workers and the values, knowledge and skills required for the work. At an international level, there is a definition of social work, international standards for practice and a statement of ethical principles (International Federation of Social Workers and International Association of Schools of Social Work 2000, 2004a, 2004b). The international definition of social work (agreed in 2000, under review in 2010–11) is as follows:

> The social work profession promotes social change, problem solving in human relationships and the empowerment and liberation of people to enhance well-being. Utilising theories of human behaviour and social systems, social work intervenes at the points where people interact with their environments. Principles of human rights and social justice are fundamental to social work.

The fact that there are internationally agreed definitions and standards may suggest that social work as practised around the world has more in common than is, in fact, the case. For how social work is practised in different countries is intrinsically linked to the nature of national and regional welfare regimes; social welfare laws and policies; the relative roles of the state, market, not-for-profit organisations and informal family and neighbourhood networks in welfare provision; prevailing cultural and religious norms about the family, gender, childhood and old age; and the value placed on equity, equality, individual and collective rights and responsibilities. This is clearly demonstrated by cases in this book. For example, Case 5.1 from Iran shows how Islamic law is embedded in the state provision of social care and influences how young women are treated in residential centres. Case 6.3 from Finland illustrates how the traditionally strong welfare state has supported care for the elderly, but this is now threatened as services are cut and privatised.

The influence of these sharp variations in the contexts in which social work is practised is especially apparent in accounts of practitioners from one country working in another. Case 3.3 is written by a Dutch social work student working in Vietnam. She questions the standard practice amongst Vietnamese physiotherapists of not discussing with service users the severity of their health problems. This very quickly leads us into the territory of ethics – raising questions about people's rights to know the truth about their medical conditions, the circumstances in which health and social care professionals should protect individuals and families from the full truth and how much weight to give to prevailing cultural norms in cases like this.

Ethics

In English we use the term 'ethics' when talking about norms and standards relating to how people should treat each other, what actions are right or wrong and which qualities of character are good or bad. It is a confusing term, as it has both a plural and a singular sense.

In its plural sense, 'ethics' is used to refer to norms or standards relating to right/wrong conduct or good/bad qualities of character. For example, we might say of someone that 'her ethics *are* very narrow'. Sometimes we use the term 'morals' to mean the same as 'ethics' in the plural sense.

'Ethics' in its singular sense refers to a set of norms, a theoretical system (e.g., Kantian ethics) or a subject area that covers norms of right/wrong conduct and qualities of good/bad character. In this sense, the term 'ethics' may be used interchangeably with 'moral philosophy'. Sometimes we use the term 'morality' to mean the same as ethics in the singular sense.

A further complication is added by the fact that the terms 'morals' and 'morality' are often used to mean the same as 'ethics' (plural) and 'ethics' (singular). However, some theorists make a distinction between morals as externally imposed normative standards or prevailing societal norms, and ethics as internally generated (personal) norms. In this book we do not make this distinction, and use the terms ethics and morals interchangeably.

In some languages there is apparently no *direct* equivalent of the term 'ethics'. Gyekye (2010) gives the example of sub-Saharan African languages. This does not mean, however, that there are no normative concepts of right and wrong conduct or good and bad character in those languages and societies. But it does mean that these facets of human existence and behaviour are conceptualised in different ways. The construction of 'ethics' as a discrete area of study, and the separation of the ethical from the practical, technical, political, cultural and religious dimensions of life is perhaps more commonly understood and accepted in the global North and West than in the South and East. On the other hand, in all parts of the world there is a recognisable normative discourse covering questions such as: 'What kinds of people should we be?' 'What kinds of lives should we live?' and 'How should we act?' The questions are recognisable, although the answers given will vary enormously between different societies, as will the extent to which the answers are inextricably linked with culture, religion and political ideology.

In this book we generally use the term 'ethics' in its singular sense to refer to a subject area that encompasses right/wrong actions (conduct), good/bad qualities of character and normative aspects of human relationships. This characterisation of ethics is deliberately broad and inclusive. For in the global South and Eastern parts of the world, and amongst some indigenous peoples (such as Native Americans or Aboriginals in Australia), normative evaluations traditionally tend to start with a focus on people's moral character ('she is a good person'; 'he is dishonest'). Judgements about actions would be framed in terms of character ('that was the act of a dishonest person'). In modern Western and Northern contexts, especially in professional ethics, the starting point is very often actions. Good/bad character would be explained in terms of right/wrong actions. These are, of course, gross generalisations. There are Eastern philosophies that place emphasis on action-based norms, and there are Western moral philosophers who argue for the primacy of character in everyday life.

Whilst the use of the term 'ethics' may leave us open to accusations of Western and Northern imperialism (as with the human rights discourse of the United Nations declarations), we wish to use the term in a broad, inclusive and critical sense. We acknowledge, however, that 'ethics' is a construction that may have more meaning in some parts of the world than others. In a social work context, just as theories, models and practices of social work have been exported from the global North and West to the South and East, so the concept of social work ethics as a separate area of study and practice is also being exported. So it will be very important for academics and practitioners across the world to take a critical approach to the subject area itself (considering what constitutes the domain of the ethical) as well as the content of this subject area (Western conceptions of individual rights, confidentiality, privacy and non-discrimination). In the next section we will consider some examples of theoretical approaches to ethics, which are often included in the largely Western literature on ethics in social work.

Theoretical and methodological approaches to ethics

Moral philosophers and ethicists have developed many different theories about the nature of the good life, what counts as human flourishing, right and wrong conduct, good and bad qualities of character. These competing ethical theories are outlined in many introductory texts on moral philosophy and in textbooks on social work ethics (Banks 2006; Boss 1998; Gray and Webb 2010; Rachels 2003; Reamer 1990). Therefore it is not our intention to go into detail here. However, we will offer a brief overview of different theoretical approaches to ethics, to give the reader a conceptual framework within which to locate the cases in the book, if desired. Further discussion of different ethical theories is also offered in some of the introductions to the chapters in this book.

Principle-based ethics

Until recently, modern Western literature on professional ethics has tended to focus on identifying and describing general and universal principles that can be used to guide ethical conduct. Reamer (introduction to Chapter 4 in this volume) describes two different schools of thought: deontological (duty-based) ethics, often associated with the eighteenth-century German philosopher Kant; and teleological (consequentialist) ethics, often associated with the nineteenth-century British utilitarians Bentham and Mill. Deontological or Kantian ethics is based on the ultimate principle of respect for persons as rational and self-determining beings. Any action which fails to accord respect to each individual person (such as lying) is wrong, regardless of whether it may produce good consequences. Utilitarian or consequentialist ethics, on the other hand, judges the rightness and wrongness of an action according to whether it produces a greater or lesser balance of beneficial over harmful consequences for the greatest number of people. According to utilitarianism, it might be regarded as morally right to lie, if lying resulted in a good outcome (saving life or bringing a lot of pleasure).

These two schools of thought are clearly in opposition, if the aim is to develop a comprehensive ethical theory based on a key foundational ethical principle. However, in everyday life, and in professional practice, principles that promote respect for individual choices and rights are equally as important as principles that promote good outcomes for individuals and society. Statements of ethical principles and codes of ethics for social work contain both these types of principles. Arguably some of our biggest ethical dilemmas and difficulties are in deciding when to compromise respect for an individual's right to freedom of choice and action in order to promote what is considered to be their greater good or the greater good of others or society in general.

According to principle-based approaches to ethics, ethical decision-making is a rational process that involves applying general principles to particular cases. The decision-maker should treat all similar cases in a similar way, as impartially and objectively as possible.

Character- and relationship-based approaches to ethics

There are alternative theoretical approaches to ethics that start with particular people and the situations in which they find themselves. We can call these approaches character- and relationship-based approaches to ethics. Virtue ethics, for example, focuses on the qualities of character of the moral agent, and asks not 'What should I do?' but 'What kind of person should I be?' and 'What would a good person do in this situation?' (Banks and Gallagher 2008; Swanton 2003). A focus on the development of good qualities of character can be found in many ancient Eastern religious teachings, including the works of Confucius, Mencius and Buddhist texts (Harvey 2000; Wong 2008). According to Gyekye (2010), character also forms the basis of African ethics. In Western philosophy, virtue ethics is traditionally associated with Aristotle (the ancient Greek philosopher), with later developments by Christian religious philosophers Aquinas and Augustine. After a period of decline in popularity, virtue ethics has recently undergone a revival in Western ethics, as a complement to or replacement for the more abstract, principle-based approaches to ethics.

Other situated approaches to ethics include the ethics of care (as discussed by Philippart in Chapter 2; see also Held 2006; Noddings 2002; Tronto 1993), which focuses on the relationships between people and the particular responsibilities inherent in special relationships (like mother and child); and the ethics of proximity, based on the responsibilities experienced in the face-to-face encounter between one person and another (Levinas 1989; Vetlesen 1997). The emphasis on relationships and responsibilities brings these approaches to ethics much closer to those that are more prevalent in the global South, where the individual is defined in relationship with others. Here much less emphasis is placed on the individual, or the relationships between individuals per se, but rather the focus is on the community (communitarian ethics), seeking solidarity, harmony and the common good (Graham 2002; Gyekye 2010).

Narrative and case-based ethics

Approaches to ethics that give primacy to character, relationships and communities very often also make use of stories as a methodology. Hilde Lindemann Nelson (1997) outlines a number of ways stories are used in ethics: to heighten moral perception and sensitivity; to promote moral education; to provide ethical justification; to define one's moral identity through telling stories and accounts; and to make ethical evaluations through comparing stories. The term 'narrative ethics' refers to a cluster of methodologies that use stories, rather than to a theoretical approach to ethics as such. Although some ethicists who have developed narrative approaches take phenomenological, social constructionist or hermeneutical perspectives (focusing on how people describe experiences, construct themselves through their stories and interpret stories as texts), many do not.

'Casuistry' or case-based ethical reasoning (Jonsen and Toulmin 1988) is sometimes grouped under the heading of 'narrative ethics', but it is very often regarded as a distinctive approach in its own right (a revival of a medieval Christian practice of providing moral guidance in particular situations). Rather than starting with an ethical theory, casuistry begins with particular cases, taking into account the specific circumstances of each case in deciding what an ethically correct response might be. It works by taking a paradigm case, which is relatively straightforward and about which most people would agree in their ethical evaluations, and then compares the case at hand with the paradigm case in order to determine differences and similarities. This is analogous to the kind of approach taken in legal reasoning, and requires skills in determining the morally relevant features of cases and in creating taxonomies of types of cases and issues. Casuistry is not a normative theory (prescribing what is good or bad), but more like a method for making ethical assessments and decisions. In case-based ethics 'moral reasoning' plays a crucial role. 'Reasoning' in this sense includes the use of moral intuition and practical wisdom and is not the same as rationality based on abstract principles (Toulmin 2001).

Given the international content of this book, this approach to ethical evaluation is helpful in that it starts with the case and advocates pursuing a detailed and careful analysis. Sometimes people who espouse very different ethical and religious values may come to agreement about what should be done in a particular case, by focusing on the details of the case. Their differences emerge when they come to justify their ethical evaluations with reference to different values or theories. In arguing for the efficacy of casuistry, Jonsen and Toulmin (1988: 16–19) give an example from their experience of a national commission on the protection of human subjects in research in the USA. They claim that whilst commissioners did not agree on a set of established universal ethical principles, they shared a common perception of what was at stake in particular cases. Jonsen and Toulmin's account is disputed by Beauchamp and Childress (1994), who claim that transcripts of the commission's deliberations show a constant movement back and forth between case and principle. Nevertheless, we would argue that analysis of cases is a very fruitful way to proceed in exploring ethical issues internationally, in contexts where very different theoretical approaches might be held. Case-based analysis can help us refine, question and develop our deeply-held ethical values. As Appiah (2007: 71) comments: 'we can agree about what to do in most cases, without agreeing about why it is right'.

Table 1.1 (adapted from Banks and Nøhr 2003: 12, with the addition of communitarian, narrative and case-based ethics) offers a brief overview of the key features of several of these different approaches to ethics, as they might be applied in social work.

Table 1.1 Some approaches to social work ethics

I Principle-based ethics (ethical theories)

a) 'Kantian' principles, for example:
    • respect for persons as rational, self-determining beings;
    • impartiality and consistency in choice and action . . .

b) Utilitarian principles, for example:
    • promotion of welfare/goods;
    • just distribution of welfare/goods . . .

II Character- and relationship-based ethics (theoretical approaches)

c) Virtue ethics – development of character/virtues/excellences, such as:
    • honesty;
    • compassion;
    • integrity . . .

d) Ethics of care – importance of particular relationships, involving:
    • care;
    • attentiveness;
    • responsibility . . .

e) Communitarian ethics – the primacy of community:
    • solidarity;
    • harmony;
    • inter-connectedness . . .

III Narrative and case-based ethics (methodologies)

f) Narrative ethics – collection of approaches that value and use stories:
    • listening to/reading stories to sharpen moral sensibilities;
    • telling stories to define and develop one's identity;
    • invoking stories as moral explanation . . .

g) Casuistry – analysis of cases as a starting point, with a focus on:
    • specific circumstances of the case
    • paradigm cases
    • categorisation and comparison of cases . . .

Adapted from Banks and Nøhr 2003.

Ethics as universal and particular

Although these many different ways of theorising about ethics, analysing cases and making ethical decisions may seem (and are sometimes presented by their proponents as) mutually exclusive, in fact they can usefully be regarded as complementary. The idea of impartial principles of fairness and universally held rights and freedoms is an important way of looking at how people should be treated, especially in professional and international contexts. Principles provide a benchmark against which to assess decisions, actions and policies and highlight unjustified differences in treatment based on favouritism, prejudice, oppressive use of power and unfair legal, social and cultural laws, customs and norms. The language of universal human rights, as found in the United Nations declarations and conventions, is a permanent reminder that cultures, religions and customs cannot be accepted and respected uncritically, but must be questioned and challenged, as Briskman and Pemán argue in the introduction to Chapter 3.

However, principle-based approaches do not capture all dimensions of what might be regarded as ethically important features of situations, especially in parts of the world or cultures where individual rights and freedoms have less prominence than family, group, tribe or community relationships and responsibilities. People's motives, character and emotions are also important, as are their particular relationships and responsibilities to each other and within their communities. Careful examination of specific features of each case or situation is vital, as is the ability to recognise morally relevant issues, to compare with other cases and to test against commonly accepted principles and rules. This capacity or quality is what Aristotle termed 'phronesis' or 'practical wisdom'. It is a quality that needs to be nurtured and developed, through working alongside experienced role models or teachers, and entails the ability to notice, pay attention and see morally relevant features of situations (Banks and Gallagher 2008).

If we take the example of Case 3.3, about the Dutch student in Vietnam, she refers to ethical principles she has learnt in the Netherlands, which stress the rights of patients and service users to information about their medical conditions and prognoses. Yet she is also aware of the cultural norms in Vietnam and the lack of experience and competence of the physiotherapists in breaking bad news. She engages in a discussion with the Vietnamese physiotherapists in an attempt to understand their perspectives and share her views with them. We could ask the question: Is the behaviour of the physiotherapists ethically right? The Dutch student's answer is that it is not, if we judge it by the standards she has learnt in the Netherlands. But by the standards operating in Vietnam, possibly it is right. Yet she does not use this experience to then go on to argue for ethical relativism based on cultural differences between the Netherlands and Vietnam. Rather, she uses the opportunity to reflect. Experience of this situation might cause her to identify some of her taken-for-granted assumptions and values (about individuals' and families' rights to information and choice), which turn out not to be as universally accepted as she might have expected. Equally she engages in conversation with the physiotherapists in order to establish how robust their taken-for-granted assumptions and values are. We do not know how things turned out in this hospital after the student left, but we might hope that both parties had learnt from each other and might slightly adjust their practices, or think more critically about what they were doing and why. For the Dutch student working in multicultural contexts in the Netherlands, she may reconsider how she approaches her work with service users of different ethnic backgrounds.

Possibilities for a global ethics?

The reflections of the Dutch student in Vietnam (Case 3.3) did not lead her to ethical relativism. Nor did she reach for universal standards of ethics generally or for social work. Some authors of cases and commentators do, however, refer to international benchmarks – for example, reference is made to the UN Convention on the Rights of the Child in Case 5.2 about rights to health care in Peru. To what extent are these international standards helpful in resolving ethical problems in local or international contexts?

United Nations declarations and conventions

The United Nations declarations and conventions (for example, those on human rights and the rights of the child, United Nations 1948; 1989) are attempts to develop a worldwide consensus on minimally accepted standards for how human beings (including peoples and communities) should treat each other and be treated by regimes and institutions. These are framed in terms of principles of action (what nation states should do) based on 'human rights' (the valid claims people have simply in virtue of being human). However, this language and way of thinking in terms of principles and rights is not the natural ethical language of many societies in the global South and East, where notions of people's character, their relationships with each other and to their communities might be more predominant. The language of principles and rights is not only a foreign imposition, it is also inevitably very abstract and general (as it is applicable to all people and in all places), hence is open to wide interpretation in its implementation (see Briskman and Pemán's introduction to Chapter 3).

Despite these challenges, the UN declarations and conventions are widely accepted in many (but by no means all) countries as providing an imperfect but useful global set of standards. They can be used to challenge particular instances of inhumane or unfair treatment as well as offering a critique of hierarchical, oppressive power structures or the subjugation of women and particular classes and castes, for example. There have been several recent attempts to adapt or develop the idea of human rights in different religious and regional contexts, as evidenced by the *Universal Islamic Declaration of Human Rights* (1980) and the *Asian Human Rights Charter* (1998), reproduced in Kymlicka and Sullivan (2007). In locating and specifying human rights in particular contexts, of course, their universal character is changed. However, the fact that the concept of human rights is being accepted and implemented in these religious and cultural contexts suggests that it has some meaning and usefulness. It also helps us to realise that the concept of international human rights belongs to a specially constructed language designed to promote international dialogue and should not be equated with that of 'individual rights' in Western liberal theory. Feinberg (1973) suggests that the use of the term 'human rights' in the UN declarations and conventions is a 'special manifesto sense of right' that identifies basic needs with rights and urges on the world community that all basic human needs should be regarded as claims worthy of serious consideration. Many alternatives to human rights as a focus for minimal international standards for treatment of people, cultures and environments have been suggested, including those starting from basic needs or human capabilities (Nussbaum 2000; Sen 1993). None of these alternatives, however, is uncontroversial.

Kymlicka (2007) suggests we should regard global ethics as a two-level phenomenon. On one level it comprises a self-standing international discourse (such as that of human rights) defining a set of minimum standards agreeable to all. At the second level there is a range of ethical traditions each of which has its own account of what is needed over and above human rights. He argues that any coming together at the second level will be the outcome of a slow process of learning and mutual exchange. Arguably, social work can also be viewed on two levels. On one level, it is an international social movement, sharing a global language and standards and concerned to work for social justice worldwide. At another level it is a professional practice necessarily rooted in particular nation-states, cultures, legal and policy frameworks. This way of looking at social work may help us understand the purpose and format of the international statement on ethics in social work.

The international statement on ethics in social work

The international statement on ethics in social work (IFSW and IASSW 2004a) embodies both these senses of social work and aims to contribute to dialogue about values, practices and ideals across boundaries. The language and concepts in this document encounter the same problems as those of the UN declarations, in that they are abstract and open to interpretation, whilst at the same time they can be accused of Northern and Western bias. For the document features concepts that are arguably less relevant or familiar in the global South, such as the rights of individuals, the importance of individual privacy and confidentiality and non-discrimination on grounds of gender, ethnicity, sexual identity, and so on. In many countries, the individual is not regarded as a primary holder of rights with an identity distinct from family, tribe or community. In some countries it is legally and culturally accepted that members of certain groups (for example, women, people of particular classes or castes, or those who are lesbian, gay or bisexual) are systematically treated less favourably than other people. In other countries such negative discrimination is legally prohibited, although this does not mean that it does not occur.

However, the work that goes into development of international statements of principles and standards (which involves consultation and negotiation between representatives from different countries) and their acceptance and publication play an important role in creating an international language in which to talk about social work and to engage in debates about the relevance, meaning and importance of key concepts and principles (such as human rights or non-discrimination). It gives participants in the debates a chance to question the values, attitudes and practices in their own countries, to reflect on how far to go in terms of accepting or respecting cultural and religious differences in their own and other countries and on what issues to take a stand and hold firm, regardless of law, religion or culture.

There are no easy answers to these questions, as many of the cases in this book demonstrate – showing social workers struggling to define and maintain professional integrity often in the face of bureaucratic, punitive and oppressive regimes. However, the cases in this book are so varied, and the commentaries are written from so many different theoretical, cultural and practical perspectives, that the book provides the ideal opportunity for students, practitioners and academics to engage in case-based reasoning, to compare and contrast different cases and responses to cases, to explore the usefulness of different theoretical perspectives and to engage in international dialogue with the cases and commentaries as well as with their colleagues. Hopefully, reflection on the issues raised by the book may help us in our journey towards a 'rooted cosmopolitanism', to use Appiah's (2007) phrase. As Appiah (ibid.: 73) comments: 'when it comes to change, what moves people is often not an argument from principle, not a long discussion about values, but just a gradually acquired new way of seeing things'.

Cases

The concept of the 'case' is central to social work – and indeed to many professions, such as law and medicine. A 'case' is more than just an individual service user, family, client, or patient; it is a constructed compilation of people, actions, events and circumstances, including partial life histories and biographies. Although 'constructed' and partial (that is, a selected assemblage of relevant features), a professional case is continually developing and unfolding until it is 'closed'. The 'professional case' in social work and other professions has both similarities with and differences from the 'case example' or 'case study' used in teaching or textbooks. The 'case example' is often a concise overview of, or a particular episode from, a 'professional case', designed to illustrate certain points (for example, good or bad practice, difficulties or dilemmas). Alternatively, a case example might just be an account of an episode from practice unrelated to an identifiable 'professional case'. A case example is an abstraction and an ordering of material from a much bigger assemblage. Strictly speaking, the 'cases' in this book are 'case examples', which fall into the more specific category of 'ethics cases'.

Ethics cases

What makes the cases in this book 'ethics cases'? The answer lies in the purpose for which they were written, the way they are interpreted by commentators and readers and the kinds of questions asked about them.

All the authors of the cases knew they were writing for a book on ethics. Some authors help the reader by highlighting what they see as the ethical dimensions of their accounts. They may refer to a 'dilemma' and identify available choices. They may invite the reader to consider which choice is preferable (leaving the ending of the case 'open') or tell the reader what decision was made and why (thus closing the ending of the case). For example, Case 2.4 ends with a social work student asking a question about whether she should have to reveal her lesbian identity to her work colleagues. We do not know what happened next, so the reader is, in effect, invited to consider what the student could or should have done. Case 2.3 concerns a Lithuanian student's dilemma about whether to accept a gift. The author of the case tells us that the student decided to take the gift, but then invites the reader to reflect on whether this was the right decision or not. These cases exhibit some of the features of traditional ethics cases (Chambers 1997): they involve a protagonist (a central person) making a difficult decision, in which some ethical issues are at stake. These ethical issues might be infringements of, or conflicts between, the rights, interests and/or needs of individuals and groups; or they might be about matters of fairness in distribution of time and services.

Other cases are simply accounts of practice, sometimes involving ethical transgressions, with no explicit decision-making or choice identified. Examples of such cases are 5.1 (a report about how care staff treated young women in Iran, including the use of deception by a social worker) and 6.3 (an account of the difficulties experienced by a woman in arranging care for her elderly mother in Finland). Although these cases are not framed in terms of the choices or decisions made, there is nevertheless an implicit invitation to the reader to consider some questions: What went wrong here and why? How could people have behaved or responded differently? How could institutions be better managed or organised to enable ethical behaviour of staff and good outcomes for service users? Such accounts of practice give more scope to readers or teachers themselves to do the ethical analysis and interpretation of the case: to identify the ethical issues; to consider hypothetical scenarios (what might have happened if . . .); and to explore contextual features of practice that influence how social workers view their work, including constraints on action.

In this book we have a broad understanding of what counts as an ethics case, which includes:

1   *Accounts of dilemmas or difficult ethical choices*, with the reader being invited to suggest a decision or course of action, or to evaluate the decision or action actually taken.
2   *Accounts of situations or series of events* that explicitly or implicitly raise ethical issues.

Shorter invented ethics cases

A common format for cases given in textbooks and used in teaching is the short case of one or two paragraphs. The case may be invented, or rewritten from students' and practitioners' accounts. In our early work with students in the European Social Ethics Project we used cases like this (Banks and Nyboe 2003). Few contextual details were given and the cases were generally not located in place and time. We deliberately constructed the cases to highlight unresolved ethical conflicts or dilemmas. They would usually end with questions – inviting the reader to suggest what course of action should be taken and hence resolve the conflict or dilemma. These cases were of type 1 mentioned above. The following example is of a short ethics case that was created by a Danish teacher, on the basis of similar stories known from practice.

> A young woman, Connie, aged 24, lives in an institution for people with learning disabilities (mentally disabled people). Connie is generally quite reserved and shy, but she has had some short, very violent and self-destructive fits. On one occasion she cut herself in the abdomen with a pair of scissors. After this event the staff tried to teach her to masturbate. Her self-destructive fits disappeared when she got into a sexual relationship with a young man at the institution. About six months ago she began a relationship with a 43-year-old man (also with learning disabilities) whom she met at the local day centre. At this time she was taking the contraceptive pill, but she has now stopped. This man is well known to the staff as he has had relationships with several female residents and has infected two of them, as well as Connie, with venereal disease. Connie has just met the man again and has told the staff that they are engaged to be married. Staff members have tried several times to discuss the issue of possible pregnancy, the advantage of using contraception and eventually getting sterilised, but Connie is not interested in their opinion. Last time they discussed it, Connie told the worker in a provocative voice that she thought it would be cool to have a little doll-baby. She has just announced that her boyfriend is coming to see her on Saturday and that he is going to stay overnight. What should the staff do?

Short, invented ethics cases like this can be very useful in teaching professional ethics in that they encourage students to think through the ethical issues involved in difficult situations. However, as Chambers (1997) points out, the construction of ethics cases in this way tends to encourage readers to analyse events, choices and actions in terms of impersonal and impartial principles and rules. This is because the case gives few details of the context in which the action takes place, the character or motives of the people involved, their past histories and relationships, or their hopes and fears. So in this case about Connie, the reader may frame the ethical issues in terms of a choice of action in which, perhaps, the right of Connie to make her own decisions is weighed against the principle of protecting Connie from future harm.

This kind of case encourages readers to make an analysis in terms of principle-based approaches to ethics (deontological or Kantian principles of respect for persons and consequentialist or utilitarian principles about promoting human welfare). However, in understanding the issues involved in a case and coming to a decision, it is also important to consider the character and motives of the particular people involved (virtue ethicists would advocate this) and the nature of the relationships they have with each other (people espousing an ethics of care or communitarian ethics would argue this). Furthermore, if we are to undertake a meaningful analysis and categorisation of this case and compare it with others, we need to know more details, including when and where it took place (a casuist might suggest this). This implies that shorter cases like the one about Connie have some limitations.

Longer real-life ethics cases

This experience led us to seek longer cases in more varied formats for this book. Essentially we were seeking reflective accounts of real-life practice that had an ethical dimension. We did not require that the cases should necessarily feature dilemmas or difficult choices. Indeed, some of the cases we received were simply accounts of events or situations (perhaps involving an implicit or explicit transgression or the taking on of an uncomfortable role). We were keen to encourage first-person accounts that might include descriptions of feelings, hopes and fears. We were also concerned to locate the cases in time and place, including the policy and legal contexts, if relevant.

The inclusion of some background information about the organisation of social work in a particular country, relevant laws, policies and so on and some reflections by the authors, helps contextualise the cases. Inevitably a case can never include all the information that a reader might require to understand fully the circumstances, constraints and possibilities of the situation. Sometimes students comment, quite rightly, that they cannot say what they would do or would have done in relation to a particular case, as they do not have enough information. For example, students in Iceland may say that they find it hard to comment on the handling of the instance of child abuse in East Jerusalem outlined in Case 6.4, as they do not know enough about the situation in the Occupied Palestinian Territories, how social workers operate there and what support and supervision they have.

This is a very valid point. However, this lack of information should not prevent students from analysing or discussing the case. Rather, the further information required to understand the case better can be turned into a series of questions, which can form part of the analysis of the case. Indeed, one of the questions students can be asked to consider in analysing a case is: What further information would you need in order to understand this case/resolve the dilemma posed? Part of the case analysis might involve asking students to undertake some research about social work in Palestine. In some cases, authors give references to background information – for example, in Case 4.2, about a young man in hospital waiting for a transplant, reference is made to protocols for organ transplants in the UK; in Case 6.1, about how refugees are treated in Australia, a reference is given to the People's Inquiry on this topic. These documents can be consulted, and comparisons made with the situation in the students' own countries. Amy Chow does this in her commentary on Case 4.2 when she discusses how transplants are organised in her own region, Hong Kong, China. In Chapter 7 we offer further ideas for a number of exercises for working with cases and commentaries.

Varieties of cases in the book

We gave all contributors some general guidelines for writing a case (similar to those outlined in Exercise VI in Chapter 7). We requested further information and made revisions to many of the cases received. Nevertheless, there is a great variety of different types of case in this book. The cases vary both in terms of their content and format.

Regarding the content of the cases, the countries in which the cases are set range from Europe through the Americas to various parts of the Middle East, Asia, Africa and Australia. The cases come from countries where social work is relatively new, or is being redeveloped (such as Vietnam and China), to countries where professional social work is well established (for example, Denmark and the USA). The practice context in which the cases are set is also varied – from social education work, youth work and hospital social work, to social work in a police station, disaster relief settings, an immigration detention centre, government social welfare offices and situations of armed conflict. The cases focus on a range of service user groups, including: children; women; families; asylum seekers; young people; older people; people with psychiatric problems; people who have committed crimes; a gypsy community; and people with terminal illnesses. The types of practice issues covered range from child sexual abuse, through adoption to social work research. The ethical issues covered are wide ranging – for example: questions about how to challenge poor or unethical practice; dilemmas about whether to withhold information from service users 'for their own good'; and debates about when it is right to 'bend' rules or policies to achieve a good outcome.

In terms of format, some cases are longer and more detailed than others. The endings of some cases are open, whilst the endings of others are closed. Some cases are told in the first person ('I did this . . .'), while the majority are told in the third person (He/she/they did that . . .'). Many of the cases told in the third person were nevertheless written, or co-authored, by someone who plays a central role in the case. The use of the third person is a way of distancing the author from the case, perhaps protecting their identity. However, a few of the cases written in the third person were written by people who were genuine observers, and were reporting on events/actions in which they did not play a leading role. Several of the cases, whilst based on real-life situations, have been slightly altered in order to maintain the anonymity of the social workers and service users.

Table 1.2 at the end of this chapter offers an overview of the cases in the book, in order to help the reader see at a glance the range of issues covered and formats used. This may help in selecting cases for discussion and study. They have been categorised according to the country in which the cases are set, and the following criteria:

- **Practice focus** – what practice issues are covered in the case (e.g., social work research, disaster relief, adoption)?
- **Ethical issues/concepts** – what are the key ethical issues covered in the case (e.g., ethical responsibilities of researchers, social workers' responses to bad practice, discrimination on the basis of sexual identity)?
- **Narrator's focus** – who is the protagonist (the person, group or organisation from whose perspective the case is told, or whose actions and deliberations feature in the foreground of the case)? Is the case told in the first person ('I did this') or third person ('she/he/they did that')?
- **Open/closed** – is the case open-ended (we do not know what happened in the end) or closed (an ending is given)?

Commentaries

The commentators were asked to offer their perspectives on the cases. The instructions for the commentators were broadly similar to those outlined in Chapter 7, Exercise II. The style and content of the commentaries varies as much as the cases. Very often two commentators from different countries make very similar points about a case – but perhaps from different perspectives or using different concepts and language. Sometimes they highlight different aspects of a case and occasionally they may present contradictory interpretations or recommendations. It can be just as interesting and illuminating to study and compare the commentaries as it is to study the cases.

The commentaries exemplify a range of ways of responding to a case, including the following:

- Identification of the key ethical and practical issues in the case ('This is a case about . . .').
- Interpretation of the case in the light of ethical theories, concepts, guidelines or codes.
- The relationship of the case to relevant laws, declarations, policies or practice guidelines.
- The relationship of the case to the commentator's own experience, country, laws, policies, ethical or cultural norms.
- Recommendations for action or resolution of problems or dilemmas.
- Raising of further questions.

Interestingly, not very many commentators systematically analyse and interpret the cases with direct reference to one or more ethical theories. Vivienne Bozalek is one of the few to do this: she analyses Case 4.3 in terms of the capabilities approach and gendered injustice. However, many commentators do make reference to ethical concepts and principles (informed consent, privacy, discrimination, rights, responsibilities, honesty), even if they do not articulate a full-blown ethical theory. There may be a number of reasons for the lack of reference to ethical theories, including the fact that the commentaries are short, hence there is little space in which to do justice to a complex theoretical position. The commentators were not asked to do this; and commentators were not necessarily selected for their expertise in theoretical ethics. It can also seem rather contrived simply to fit a case into a theoretical framework. However, perhaps the way the commentaries are written (even by those who are professional philosophers and who have expertise in professional ethics) tells us something about the usefulness of ethical theories for practical ethics. Whilst awareness of different ethical theories may give us some resources to see different aspects of a case (respect for rights, consequences, character, responsibilities and relationships), ultimately it is what Jonsen (1996) calls 'the morally appreciated circumstances' of each case on which the commentators focus.

Concluding comments

In Chapter 7 we outline some of the ways in which the materials presented in this book can be used, and we are sure there are many more possibilities. The richness of the cases and commentaries will draw readers and discussants in new and surprising directions. Although there is no substitute for real-life international discussions where the authors of the cases can answer back in person, we nevertheless hope that the complexity and diversity of the situations and views expressed in this book will challenge our certainties and complacency. We hope the book will contribute to the promotion of greater international understanding and greater commitment to resist injustice amongst social workers worldwide and to work for transformatory change in their workplaces, communities and societies. Through this book, and the conversations that emerge from it, we hope in some small measure to stimulate what a Portuguese student reported as a result of her participation in an international exchange programme organised by the European Social Ethics Project (Liebing and Møller 2003: 156):

> I feel that I have become a rich woman now. When I come home, I shall still have this group inside my head. After this I shall not act immediately, when I meet a difficult situation or an ethical dilemma in my practice. Instead I shall discuss the situation with my group inside my head. I shall say to myself: What would the Finnish student say or do in this situation? And what would be the point of view of the Belgian student? How would the Danish student react to this problem, and what would the German student consider important? In this way I would be able to think of many important aspects and many different alternatives, before I decide how to act in practice.

Table 1.2 Overview of cases

Case	Country where case is set	Practice focus	Key ethical issues	Narrator's perspective	Open ended/ closed
2.1	China	Social work in post-disaster situations. Work with young people in a school.	How to respond to incompetent and unethical practice.	A social work team. 3rd person.	Open
2.2	Botswana	Social work in a police station. Sexual abuse and violence between mother and son.	How a social work intern responds to an account of sexual abuse and violence in a family.	Observer of an intern and a young man. 3rd person.	Open
2.3	Lithuania	Social work with refuges. Chechenian families.	Whether to accept a gift.	Academic about a student. 3rd person.	Closed, but questions raised
2.4	UK	Residential child care. Professional relationships.	Too close relationships with service users. Whether to come out as a lesbian.	Social work student. 3rd person.	Open
3.1	USA	Social work in a psychiatric hospital. A man diagnosed with bipolar disorder.	Balancing respect for choice and the coercion of a patient/ service user. Clash of values between medical staff and social worker.	Social worker. 1st person.	Closed

Table 1.2 Continued

Case	Country where case is set	Practice focus	Key ethical issues	Narrator's perspective	Open ended/closed
3.2	Sweden	Residential care for elderly people. Caring for a man with Alzheimer's disease.	Balancing respect for choice of service user with minimal competence against wishes of partner and long-term personal integrity of service user.	Staff and professional association. 3rd person.	Part 1: open; Part 2: closed
3.3	Vietnam	Rehabilitation department of a hospital. A boy with Duchenne Muscular Dystrophy.	Withholding information about a child's medical condition from a family. Clash of values between Vietnamese physiotherapists and Dutch student social worker.	Social work student. 1st person.	Closed
3.4	India	Social work research. Post-disaster situation (tsunami).	Whether and how to respond when researchers witness negative discrimination and corrupt practices.	Research team of social work academics. 3rd person.	Open
4.1	Japan	Social work in a state social welfare agency. Illegal migrant and child.	Inability of social worker to treat illegal migrant fairly. Clash of social work values and values of state social welfare organisation.	Social worker. 1st person.	Closed

4.2	UK	Social work in a hospital. Young man waiting for heart and lung transplant.	Whether to withhold information from a competent patient and family. Clash of values between health care staff and social worker.	Social worker. 3rd person.	Closed
4.3	Portugal	Social education work with gypsy families. Work with a young woman on school attendance.	Balancing respect for gypsy culture with rights, wishes and welfare of young woman. Male domination.	Social educator. 3rd person.	Open
4.4	Turkey	Social work in the adoption field. Gay man wishing to adopt a child.	Balancing rights and welfare of potential adopted child with the rights of a gay man to adopt a child. Discrimination against gay people.	Social worker. 3rd person.	Closed
5.1	Iran	Residential centre and crisis intervention service for young women.	Use of deception by a social worker to obtain information. Religious and organisational restrictions on young women's choices and actions.	Impartial narrator. 3rd person.	Closed

Table 1.2 Continued

Case	Country where case is set	Practice focus	Key ethical issues	Narrator's perspective	Open ended/closed
5.2	Peru	Social work in a health insurance office. Eligibility of a child for support when the father is no longer taking responsibility.	Rights of a child. Social workers taking action to make exceptions to rules, and to create new rules to accommodate service users in genuine need.	Social worker. 1st person.	Closed
5.3	Australia	Social work in a Christian church-based mental health counselling service. Young man with schizophrenia.	Challenging poor and unethical practice of a volunteer. Conflict between social worker's professional values and loyalty to his religious faith.	Social worker. 1st person.	Closed
5.4	Denmark	School in an area of high minority ethnic population. Class of eight-year old children.	Whether it was right for school staff to handle widespread occurrence of physical punishment by parents without involving the social authorities.	Impartial narrator. 3rd person.	Closed
6.1	Australia	Social work in a refugee settlement agency.	Dilemmas regarding how to respond to inadequate and demeaning treatment of refugees (based on government policy).	Social worker. 3rd person.	Closed

6.2	Pakistan	Women's and children's NGO. Work in an area of political conflict.	How to maintain the integrity of an NGO and its values, whilst being pragmatic in working with the headmen of the Taliban. Male domination.	Organisation. 3rd person.	Closed
6.3	Finland	Care for older people. A woman with Alzheimer's disease.	The role of the welfare state in provision of services. Challenges to the dignity of service users.	Carer. 1st person.	Ongoing issue
6.4	Palestine	Social work in a school. Child sexual abuse. Work in an area of political conflict.	Protecting a child, while avoiding family shame and the involvement of Israeli authorities.	Teacher and social worker. 3rd person.	Closed
7.1	China	NGO working with poor children.	Dilemma regarding whether to take money from a dubious source.	Social worker. 3rd person.	Open
7.2	France	Social work with illegal migrants. The role of the professional association in supporting social workers.	Maintenance of professional secrecy by a social worker, in spite of pressure from the police.	Professional association. 3rd person.	Closed

Table 1.2 Continued

Case	Country where case is set	Practice focus	Key ethical issues	Narrator's perspective	Open ended/ closed
7.3	Jamaica	Social work department in a university. Child sexual abuse.	Dilemma about whether to blow the whistle on a colleague who may be engaging in poor practice.	University Director of Field Education. 3rd person.	Open
7.4	Malaysia	Youth work by Muslim Youth Association. Young people with antisocial and criminal behaviour in a school.	Dilemma about whether to continue with a successful youth programme that involved young people spending several nights in prison as a means of deterrence.	Youth worker. 1st and 3rd person.	Closed
7.5	Spain	Social work in a shelter for homeless people.	Whether to enforce or break the rules of the shelter in relation to a particular person.	Impartial observer. 3rd person.	Open
7.6	Finland	Youth work in an open access youth house. Work with a girl with learning disabilities.	Whether to allow a young woman access to a youth house, which was beneficial for her, when her mother had banned her from attending.	Youth worker. 1st person.	Open

References

Aadland, E. (1998) *Etikk for helse- og sosialarbeidarar [Ethics for Health and Social Workers]*, Oslo: Det Norske Samlaget.

Appiah, K. (2007) *Cosmopolitanism: Ethics in a World of Strangers*, London: Penguin.

Banks, S. (2006) *Ethics and Values in Social Work*, 3rd edition, Basingstoke: Palgrave Macmillan.

—— (2008) 'Critical commentary: social work ethics', *British Journal of Social Work* 38(6): 1238–1249.

Banks, S. and Gallagher, A. (2008) *Ethics in Professional Life: Virtues for Health and Social Care*, Basingstoke: Palgrave Macmillan.

Banks, S., Hugman, R., Healy, L., Bozalek, V. and Orme, J. (2008) 'Global ethics for social work: problems and possibilities', *Ethics and Social Welfare* 2(3): 276–290.

Banks, S. and Nøhr, K. (2003) 'Introduction', in S. Banks and K. Nøhr (eds) *Teaching Practical Ethics for the Social Professions*, Copenhagen: FESET.

Banks, S. and Nyboe, N.-E. (2003) 'Writing and using cases', in S. Banks and K. Nøhr (eds) *Teaching Practical Ethics for the Social Professions*, Copenhagen: FESET.

Beauchamp, T. and Childress, J. (1994) *Principles of Biomedical Ethics*, 4th edition, Oxford and New York: Oxford University Press.

Beckett, C. and Maynard, A. (2005) *Values and Ethics in Social Work: An Introduction*, Sage: London.

Boss, J. (1998) *Ethics for Life: An Interdisciplinary and Multi-Cultural Introduction*, Mountain View, CA: Mayfield.

Bowles, W., Collingridge, M., Curry, S. and Valentine, B. (2006) *Ethical Practice in Social Work: An Applied Approach*, Crow's Nest, New South Wales: Allen and Unwin.

Chambers, T. (1997) 'What to expect from an ethics case (and what it expects from you)', in H. Nelson (ed.) *Stories and Their Limits: Narrative Approaches to Bioethics*, New York and London: Routledge.

Charleton, M. (2007) *Ethics for Social Care in Ireland: Philosophy and Practice*, Dublin: Gill and Macmillan.

Congress, E., Black, P. and Strom-Gottfried, K. (eds) (2009) *Teaching Social Work Ethics and Values: A Curriculum Resource*, Alexandra, VA: Council on Social Work Education.

Cox, D. and Pawar, M. (2006) *International Social Work: Issues, Strategies and Programs*, Thousand Oaks, CA: Sage.

Dolgoff, R., Loewenberg, F. and Harrington, D. (2009) *Ethical Decisions for Social Work Practice*, 8th edition, Belmont, CA: Brooks Cole.

Feinberg, J. (1973) *Social Philosophy*, Englewood Cliffs, NJ: Prentice Hall.

Graham, M. (2002) *Social Work and African-Centred Worldviews*, Birmingham: Venture Press.

Gray, M. and Webb, S. (eds) (2010) *Ethics and Value Perspectives in Social Work*, Basingstoke: Palgrave Macmillan.

Gyekye, K. (2010) 'African ethics', *Stanford Encyclopedia of Philosophy*, http://plato.stanford.edu/entries/african-ethics/, accessed December 2010.

Harvey, P. (2000) *An Introduction to Buddhist Ethics*, Cambridge: Cambridge University Press

Healy, L. (2001) *International Social Work: Professional Action in an Interdependent World*, New York/Oxford: Oxford University Press.

—— (2007) 'Universalism and cultural relativism in social work ethics', *International Social Work* 50(1): 11–26.

Held, V. (2006) *The Ethics of Care: Personal, Political, and Global*, Oxford: Oxford University Press.

Hugman, R. (2008) 'Ethics in a world of difference', *Ethics and Social Welfare* 2(2): 118–132.

—— (2010) *Understanding International Social Work: A Critical Analysis*, Basingstoke: Palgrave Macmillan.

International Federation of Social Workers and International Association of Schools of Social Work (2000) *Definition of Social Work*: IASSW and IFSW, available at www.iassw-aiets.org.

—— (2004a) *Ethics in Social Work, Statement of Principles*, Berne: IFSW and IASSW, available at: www.ifsw.org.

—— (2004b) *Global Standards*: IASSW and IFSW, available at www.iassw-aiets.org.

Jonsen, A. (1996) 'Morally appreciated circumstances: a theoretical problem for casuistry', in L. Sumner and J. Boyle (eds) *Philosophical Perspectives on Bioethics*, Toronto: Toronto University Press.

Jonsen, A. and Toulmin, S. (1988) *The Abuse of Casuistry: A History of Moral Reasoning*, Berkeley, CA: University of California Press.

Joseph, J. and Fernandes, G. (eds) (2006) *An Enquiry into Ethical Dilemmas in Social Work*, Mumbai: College of Social Work, Nirmala Niketan.

Kymlicka, W. (2007) 'Introduction: the globalisation of ethics', in W. Sullivan and W. Kymlicka (eds) *The Globalisation of Ethics*, Cambridge: Cambridge University Press.

Kymlicka, W. and Sullivan, W. (eds) (2007) *The Globalisation of Ethics*, Cambridge: Cambridge University Press.

Levinas, E. (1989) 'Ethics as first philosophy', translated by Seán Hand, in S. Hand (ed.) *The Levinas Reader*, Oxford: Blackwell.

Liebing, A. and Møller, B. (2003) 'Teaching ethics in an international context', in S. Banks and K. Nøhr (eds) *Teaching Practical Ethics for the Social Professions*, Copenhagen: FESET.

Lingås, L. (1992) *Etikk og verdivalg i helse- og sosialfag [Ethics and the Choice of Values in Health and Social Professions]*, Oslo: Universitetsforlaget AS.

Linzer, N. (1999) *Resolving Ethical Dilemmas for Social Work Practice*, Needham Heights, MA: Allyn and Bacon.

Lyons, K., Manion, K. and Carlsen, M. (2006) *International Perspectives on Social Work*, Basingstoke: Palgrave Macmillan.

Nelson, H. L. (1997) 'Introduction: how to do things with stories', in H. L. Nelson (ed.) *Stories and Their Limits: Narrative Approaches to Bioethics*, New York and London: Routledge.

Noddings, N. (2002) *Starting at Home: Caring and Social Policy*, Berkeley and Los Angeles, CA: University of California Press.

Nussbaum, M. (2000) *Women and Human Development*, Cambridge: Cambridge University Press.

Payne, M. (2000) 'The nature of social work', in M. Davies (ed.) *The Blackwell Encyclopaedia of Social Work*, Oxford: Blackwell.

Rachels, J. (2003) *The Elements of Moral Philosophy*, 4th edition, New York: McGraw-Hill.

Reamer, F. (1990) *Ethical Dilemmas in Social Service*, 2nd edition, New York: Columbia University Press.

—— (2006) *Social Work Values and Ethics*, 3rd edition, New York: Columbia University Press.

—— (2009) *The Social Work Ethics Casebook: Cases and Commentary*, Washington: NASW Press.

Rothman, J. (2005) *From the Front Lines: Student Cases in Social Work Ethics*, Boston, MA: Pearson Education.

Rouzel, J. (1997) *Le travail d'éducateur spécialisé: éthique et pratique*, Paris: Dunod.

Sen, A. (1993) 'Capability and well-being', in M. Nussbaum and A. Sen (eds) *The Quality of Life*, Oxford: Clarendon Press.

Swanton, C. (2003) *Virtue Ethics: A Pluralistic View*, Oxford: Oxford University Press.

Toulmin, S. (2001) *Return to Reason*, Cambridge, MA: Harvard University Press.

Tronto, J. (1993) *Moral Boundaries: A Political Argument for an Ethic of Care*, London: Routledge.

United Nations (1948) *Universal Declaration of Human Rights*, www.un.org/en/documents/udhr/.

United Nations (1989) *United Nations Convention on the Rights of the Child*, www2.ohchr.org/english/law/crc.htm.

Vetlesen, A. (1997) 'Introducing an ethics of proximity', in H. Jodalen and A. Vetleson (eds) *Closeness: An Ethics*, Oslo: Scandinavian University Press.

Wong, D. (2008) 'Chinese ethics', *Stanford Encyclopedia of Philosophy*, http://plato.stanford.edu/entries/ethics-chinese/, accessed December 2010.

2 | Negotiating roles and boundaries

Introduction

FRANK PHILIPPART

What does it mean to be a professional social worker?

One of the characteristic features of the history of social work is that most social interventions, until well into the twentieth century, were carried out by well-informed volunteers (unpaid workers). The first school of social work in the world was started in Amsterdam in 1899, with others quickly following in Europe and North America, then in the 1920s and 1930s in parts of South America, Africa and Asia (Healy 2001: 21–23). At this time the work concentrated particularly on issues of poverty, hygiene and antisocial behaviour. Social work gradually began to 'professionalise' in most Western countries during the course of the twentieth century, as overall prosperity grew and governments became increasingly aware of the need to educate citizens in 'social' behaviour, to control and contain growing social problems and to introduce supportive measures to counteract the effects of economic and other material inequalities.

'Professionalisation' is usually regarded as entailing the introduction of professional education and training in higher education institutions, the production of specialist literature, the development of professional practice and the adoption of professional codes of ethics. It is also a process of gaining status and credibility for an occupational group, and has been regarded with some suspicion by certain parts of the social work community, as professionalisation is associated with exclusivity and elitism (Banks 2006: 74–77). Social work has always attracted individuals with a strong social conscience and a personal commitment to provide help and to work towards social change for the benefit of more vulnerable and disadvantaged citizens. This means that in social work a value is placed not only upon professionalism, but also upon the vocation (personal commitment or calling) and social activism of its practitioners. Case 2.1, about disaster relief following an earthquake in China, is an example of conflicting perceptions of what counts as 'good help'. Here qualified social workers observed what they regarded as incompetent and unethical practice amongst volunteer relief workers. However, because social work, along with its professional values and standards, is not currently well established or well known in China, they hesitated about whether and how to draw attention to these deficiencies.

With the achievement of social legislation, social insurance and social rights in most Western and many other societies, professional social workers became employees of social organisations, either directly employed or often subsidised by the state, and therefore required to work according to official rules and regulations. At this point social work practitioners began to experience a gap between their social commitment and ideals on the one hand, and the rules and regulations of the employing organisation on the other hand. It became characteristic for social workers to combine very different roles as part of their professional responsibilities, ranging from carer or advocate to assessor or controller.

Since social workers frequently come into close contact with service users and have access to personal information, these different roles can come into conflict with each other. For professional practitioners have obligations both to service users and also to employing organisations, which in turn have goals linked to the public interest. In cases where the personal and/or professional interests or values of social workers are in conflict with the public interests or values of organisations, social workers find themselves in uncomfortable positions. Indeed, many social workers often find it difficult to establish relationships with service users based on mutual trust, knowing that they must give warnings that certain types of information received cannot remain confidential and that assessments or reports will be made that may have unwelcome consequences.

Choosing and negotiating roles within the job

Social workers operate in a wide range of settings – from individual private practice to organisations in the private, voluntary and public sectors. The type of client-group and the kind of service the practitioner provides necessarily influences the roles adopted. In choosing and moving between the roles of carer, advocate, assessor or controller, for example, practitioners are also guided by the types of working relationships they have with the service users. These relationships can be placed on a continuum from voluntary to compulsory. In an ideal world, voluntary relationships between social workers and service users might entail service users acknowledging and understanding the problems, needs or other issues they face and knowing they cannot be solved without asking for help or working in partnership with a social professional. Service users would be prepared to talk about their issues and would be willing to explore different solutions. The initiative for the contact might come from the service users. However, in very few cases do relationships between social workers and service users meet all these criteria for voluntary engagement and consent. In most cases service users may be ambivalent, and in order to get results in terms of well-being for service users and others, social workers may exert some persuasion or pressure.

At the other extreme, involuntary service users might deny that they are experiencing problems or issues that require intervention or some kind of partnership working. They may refuse to talk with 'outsiders' about their problems and give no consideration to handling things differently. The initiative for the contact may come from others. Involuntary social work is very common in probation services, domestic violence, child protection work and mental health care, when people may constitute dangers to themselves or others. This is exemplified in Case 2.2, written from the perspective of a social work student working in a police station in Botswana.

In all cases, from voluntary to involuntary social work, it is important that social workers operate within a framework of professional ethics, in order to ensure respectful treatment of service users, fair processes and just outcomes. In cases of compulsory social work this is even more important, because the freedom of service users is, in some ways, restricted.

Professional responsibilities and duties

In most countries in the world where social work is practised there are professional associations or other bodies that have developed, and play a role in upholding, statements of values and purpose. Very often there are codes of ethics that outline the basic principles of social work and give details of the overall responsibilities and specific duties of social workers (Banks 2006: 77–102). These may sometimes be based on, or at least make reference to, the international statement on ethics in social work (IFSW and IASSW 2004). In most countries it is accepted that social workers have basic responsibilities to respect the rights and dignity of service users and to give full and sound information on the significance of the judicial framework for the working relationship. This latter point is very important, especially for involuntary service users who need to know what their rights and obligations are and what can and cannot be done within any particular judicial framework.

Ethical dilemmas arise when the personal interests of service users conflict with the professional and ethical judgements of social workers, and/or with the public need for safety and security, and/or the interests of the social work organisation to control and limit undesirable behaviour. Organisations are very often set up with the aim of working towards changing service users' behaviour so that it becomes more constructive. Many service users react negatively when serious measures are imposed upon them. Social workers may need to make ethical judgements about when they have a responsibility or moral obligation to intervene in relation to what they regard as wrongful behaviour. This might include situations when: workers get knowledge of possible harm that can be done to others; service users clearly act against the law; service users are considered a threat to public safety; service users talk about others in a disrespectful or even harmful way; service users act against the moral convictions of the worker; or service users with a different cultural background to the worker exhibit antisocial behaviour. Normally professional practitioners work, even in compulsory social work, in cooperation with service users, but they do have to decide at what point they should work against their will and without their consent.

Professional distance and professional closeness

Making judgements about where to place the boundaries between personal and professional life is a great challenge for a wide range of social care workers, youth workers and pedagogues who work in people's living environments, provide intimate care and may develop long-term relationships with service users. This is exemplified in Case 2.4, which is about a student working in a residential care home. Her co-workers judged she was developing a personal relationship with a young man that was too close.

To do the job well, social workers have to be able to understand and communicate on a social and psychological level with people of very different social and cultural backgrounds. This demands the ability to develop a degree of closeness with service users. However, it is important to distinguish this *professional* closeness from *personal* closeness. Professionals should have no personal need for closeness with particular service users. However, a degree of professional closeness is necessary to communicate with service users and to develop mutual trust and understanding in the relationship. Professional closeness entails the ability to empathise, to understand as fully as possible service users' situations, hopes, fears and desires and to respond with compassion. However, the essence of professional closeness is that it is also balanced by a certain degree of professional distance. What is meant in this context by 'professional distance' is the introduction of certain social and ethical rules and boundaries relating to the relationships between service users and professionals. Professional distance also enables social workers to intervene in historically developed, but socially and ethically unacceptable, forms and patterns of behaviour and work towards the well-being of all involved. Case 2.3 about a student wondering whether she should have accepted a gift from a service user is a good example of a practitioner who is aware of the need for some rules and boundaries, but is not sure where to locate them.

The role of a professional social worker requires an ability to balance the different sets of meanings and interests of service users, their families, neighbours and others. Social workers often find themselves in situations where they come to know personal and private information. This information may be about circumstances or activities that are potentially hazardous to other people. Yet revealing the information can also endanger the trust and closeness of the relationship with service users. Decision-making in these matters involves the making of judgements based on professionally accepted principles and rules.

The ethics of justice and care

What we have just described as 'professional distance' and 'professional closeness' can be linked to two theoretical approaches to ethics: the 'ethics of justice' and the 'ethics of care'. The 'ethics of justice' takes as its starting point a set of abstract, universal principles about how people should treat each other. The 'ethics of care', on the other hand, focuses on the unique and situated relationship between the care-giver and the recipient of care (Gilligan 1982; Noddings 1984; Sevenhuisen 1998). In day-to-day social work practice, both approaches to ethics are relevant in developing relationships with people and deciding how to act. Lohman and Raaff (2001) argue that the most important challenge for social professionals is to seek to reconcile the differences between the two ethical systems, which can be seen in the context of the discretionary space in which the worker is free to determine how to act in a specific case. In the 'ethics of justice' there is a great emphasis on principles of equality, an attitude of objectivity in addressing the other, rational thinking in considering the matter at hand, respect for universal values, duty to follow laws and obligations, respect for the autonomy and civil rights of service users and an obligation to work on behalf of service users. All these values and principles are recognised by every professional practitioner in the field. We also recognise here the ethical thinking of John Rawls (1973) and Immanuel Kant (1797/1959). This kind of ethical thinking is ingrained in modern Western societies. However, this way of thinking has disadvantages. It could be argued that it tends to lead towards a legalistic model of individual rights and duties, whereby help is given to people on the basis of rights that are acquired through a process of conflict and struggle between different interest groups and individuals.

As already mentioned, the 'ethics of care' works from a quite different set of values, including: valuing the uniqueness and difference of each person, applying relational values (such as love, care or trust), understanding people in context, starting with people's own perspectives, valuing commitment to the person in need, acknowledging dependency and working for altruistic motives. However, this approach also has its disadvantages. It can encourage a growth in dependency or even institutionalisation, it may reinforce the danger of social exclusion (by treating individuals in isolation) and there may be a lack of clarity and an arbitrariness in the nature of the help given (as it depends on unique relationships rather than universal, impartial principles and rules).

Conclusion

As the preceding discussion suggests, neither the ethics of care nor the ethics of justice are adequate on their own as approaches to understanding the ethical dimensions of practice and making ethical decisions in social work. Rather than seeing these as conflicting approaches to ethics, it could be argued that they are, in fact, complementary. In social work, as in life generally, we need to value unique relationships and commitments and offer care and compassion towards each other, at the same time as taking account of the bigger picture, guarding against unfair and preferential treatment and promoting equity (Banks 2004: 98–105).

One of the defining characteristics of professionals is the fact that they work within a discretionary space where they have a certain degree of freedom to make their own decisions on how to proceed in relation to particular cases. In this process professionals often have to negotiate demands for care, closeness and compassion with requirements for objectivity, distance and justice in distribution of time and resources. Cases 2.2, 2.3 and 2.4 in this chapter illustrate some of these negotiations in practice. In these three cases, the social work practitioners are all students reflecting on where to draw lines between personal and professional life and deliberating about what should be their proper roles in relation to particular service users. As the commentaries from experienced practitioners and academics demonstrate, there are no easy answers to these challenging questions, which require ethical sensitivity to the nuances of the particular relationships and commitments at stake, as well as a clear understanding of the principles and procedures of the profession and employing agency designed to protect service users and promote fairness.

References

Banks, S. (2004) *Ethics, Accountability and the Social Professions*, Basingstoke: Palgrave Macmillan.

Banks, S. (2006) *Ethics and Values in Social Work*, 3rd edition, Basingstoke: Palgrave Macmillan.

Gilligan, C. (1982) *In a Different Voice: Psychological Theory and Women's Development*, Cambridge, MA: Harvard University Press.

Healy, L. (2001) *International Social Work: Professional Action in an Interdependent World*, New York/Oxford: Oxford University Press.

International Federation of Social Workers and International Association of Schools of Social Work (2004) *Ethics in Social Work, Statement of Principles*, www.ifsw.org, accessed October 2010.

Kant, I. (1797) [1959 edition] *Foundations of the Metaphysics of Morals*, translated by L. W. Beck, New York: Liberal Arts Press.

Lohman, S. and Raaf, H. (2001) *In de frontlinie tussen hulp en recht [In the Frontline Between Help and Right]*, Bussum, Netherlands: Uitgeverij Coutinho.

Noddings, N. (1984) *Caring: A Feminine Approach to Ethics and Moral Education*, Berkeley and Los Angeles, CA: University of California Press.

Rawls, J. (1973) *A Theory of Justice*, Oxford: Oxford University Press.

Sevenhuisen, S. (1998) *Citizenship and the Ethics of Care: Feminist Considerations on Justice, Morality and Politics*, London: Routledge.

Case 2.1   Doing harm with a good heart: volunteer social work in a post-disaster situation in China

Introduction

This case is about voluntary social work in mainland China following the Sichuan earthquake on 12th May 2008. Many volunteers become involved in post-disaster management work. But they may not always be adequately prepared or trained to carry out what may be helpful for the disaster survivors. This is especially so in contexts where social work is less developed, and where coordination is not the call of the day. In mainland China (with the exception of Hong Kong), social work is a fledgling profession. Social work programmes were reinstated only in 1989, since all related programmes were closed in 1949 when the Communist Party took power. Most people in China are not aware of the existence of social workers nor of what they do.

The case

The magnitude 8 earthquake that ravaged Sichuan on 12th May 2008 killed 70,000, injured 375,000 and displaced 15 million people.[1] The People's Liberation Army (PLA),[2] medical personnel, teachers, and volunteers were highly recognised and respected for their contribution to the rescue work. Mainland Chinese social workers sprang into action too, though their professional knowledge and skills were not recognised by the authorities or the general public, as social work is little known about in China. Social workers were often associated as volunteers. The difficult situation was further compounded by the lack of training and the lack of experience of both unqualified volunteers and social workers.

In a school that was hit hard by the earthquake, where approximately 220 students died and more than 100 students suffered severe, disabling

---

1 See International Federation of Red Cross and Red Crescent Societies, 2008, www.reliefweb.int/rw/rwb.nsf/db900SID/EDIS-7LLLK2?OpenDocument
2 The PLA is the unified military organisation of all land, sea, strategic missile and air forces of the People's Republic of China.

injuries, the principal opened the school doors to groups offering social services to provide additional help and support for the students in need. This included a professional social work station with four newly graduated local social workers and two rehabilitation therapists. They provided a range of services, including rehabilitation social work.

The social workers and rehabilitation therapists soon found out that another volunteer group, which was affiliated to and funded by a commercial company based in another city, had also begun to provide a rehabilitation service, with rather fancy equipment and play stations. For instance, they provided a physical therapy ramp or a staircase training unit in their activity room, which actually required the presence of trained professionals when in use. However, this volunteer group did not have any professional staff, other than a volunteer who was a fresh graduate from a law school and would visit the school on a daily basis. Occasionally, other part-time volunteers of this volunteer group would come to help the students use the equipment, which actually required professional guidance.

When the social workers did a background check on the volunteer group, they soon found that the students' photos were splashed over the internet, including the personal webpage of the person in charge of the volunteer group. Some of the photos even revealed amputated body parts of the students in a graphic manner. The social workers and rehabilitation therapists were concerned about the 'service' provided by the group. If they were to approach the principal, the social workers feared that the principal might misunderstand and think that they were trying to make it difficult for the volunteer group, which might be regarded as being in competition with the social work station. The social workers wondered if they should do anything about the situation, of which the principal may or may not have been aware.

Commentary 1

ANGELA ON KEE TSUN

The Sichuan earthquake was a sorrowful and disheartening event for us all. Individuals, volunteer groups and NGOs from different parts of China and the world wanted to give a helping hand as there was much to cope with in the aftermath of the disaster. Both the newly graduated local social workers and the volunteer group were offering their resources to do what they could with a good heart.

Social work is an evaluative discipline, where social workers often need to make judgements and decisions on what is the 'right' thing to do according to the ethical codes of practice by which we all abide. Understandably, the four social work volunteers might have assumed that the volunteer group had broken the code of confidentiality by placing sensitive material on the personal webpage of the person-in-charge, including posting students' photos (some showing amputated body parts) in a graphic manner. Volunteers using rehabilitative equipment and play stations without prior training could also be seen as unethical and as failing to ensure the safety of the users. The social workers would like to have stopped these acts, which could be defined as unethical according to the ethical standards of social work.

Indeed, ethics is at the heart of social work practice. Social workers' concerns and intentions stimulate further thoughts on ethical practice. Looking at the situation through a postmodern lens, we may wish to 'question', 're-position' and 're-focus' (Bowles et al. 2006: 21) what these values and ethics are. Are we to treat these ethical principles as absolute standards, which we all follow without question? Are these ethical principles fixed discourses leaving culture and contextual factors unattended? Are professional knowledge and skills necessarily better than the local knowledge of individuals and groups? Would we want to establish a territory that differentiates professionals from non- or para-professionals?

I am curious to know whether the person-in-charge and the students might have been consulted and whether they had given informed consent to uploading the personal webpage, photos and graphic presentations. If we had been present in this situation, we could have explored the volunteer group's intentions and values in taking this course of action, and could have tried to understand more of the commitment of the person-in-charge to the service. I can imagine that in a big country like China, cyberspace is an effective platform for the dissemination of information, and a good means to attract continued attention and donors' contributions.

Before taking further action to alert the principal of the volunteer group's potentially unethical practice, the social work volunteer group discussed the issue among themselves and considered the potentially deleterious effect of approaching the school principal (since they might be seen as competing with the volunteer group). I cannot agree more with them and appreciate their mindful thoughts and responsible behaviour. Not taking such action could also have prevented them from speaking from a position of power to judge and devalue the volunteer group's service.

Apart from the ethical lens through which social workers are supposed to view things, we can make new meanings from other lenses. Perhaps it was preferable to have immediately the rehabilitative equipment and play facilities that could provide timely service, and are believed to be beneficial to people after trauma, rather than to have waited for trained professionals or for people to have been trained. Perhaps the person-in-charge, the students and even the principal would have wanted the 'real picture' (from the website) to reach the public, as they might have been aware that in China news is often screened before dissemination and the reality is only partly disclosed. Uploading of photos and graphic presentations of amputated body parts could have been one of the ways to connect people staying in Sichuan with other Chinese people (perceived as members of kin and community) and the outside world.

I could imagine some possible alternative courses of action in working for the welfare of the students, which include: (1) collaborative efforts with an equitable relationship between the two groups of relief workers; (2) collaborative work such as the social workers providing training for the volunteers on the use of the equipment; (3) dialogues between the social workers and the volunteer group so that they could learn from each other how best the students could be involved in the process and supported in life's difficult moments.

The scenario also reminds me how we can reposition ourselves: social work is a profession with values and ethical principles, which are indeed useful guides for moral behaviour and good practice. Nonetheless, these values and ethics should in no way prevent us from respecting and honouring the efforts of others. The power given to us should not block us from listening to others' words nor from working in partnership with other people/disciplines; nor should it lead us to subjugate others' voices.

Reference

Bowles, W., Collingridge, M., Curry, S. and Valentine, B. (2006) *Ethical Practice in Social Work: An Applied Approach*, Maidenhead: Open University Press.

Angela On Kee Tsun is Associate Head and Associate Professor, Department of Social Work, Hong Kong Baptist University, China.

Commentary 2

GRANT LARSON AND JULIE DROLET

This is an interesting scenario that takes place in a post-disaster situation in China, but it has parallels in other contexts where volunteers and other disciplines are involved in providing social services. Although social work is a new profession in China, similar dilemmas regarding roles and boundaries are evident in other countries where social work is well established as a profession. The ethical question in this situation focuses on the role professional social workers should play when they become aware that the services others are providing to vulnerable populations are inadequate, dangerous and perhaps an infringement of their rights. Specifically, do Chinese social workers have an ethical obligation to take their concerns outside of their own organisation, or do they respect the right of others (including volunteers) to perform necessary work in the way they (volunteers) feel is appropriate and needed? Would they be crossing a professional boundary by interfering with a service delivered by the volunteer group?

This particular ethical dilemma is complicated by the specific context in which the service is being provided. The case highlights that social work in mainland China is not well known or understood. Thus, the ethical codes and practices of the profession are likely not well understood or perhaps not even articulated in a formal sense. Also, service in this situation is being provided in a post-disaster context and it is not uncommon, in our experience, that in disaster situations, untrained and unqualified volunteers are often utilised as governmental and professional resources are limited given the magnitude of need. The 'questionable' service in this case is being provided by a commercial organisation located in the same school, but not under the auspices of the social workers' organisation. In addition, the service is being provided by volunteers, not trained professionals, so it is understandable that a volunteer organisation with a commercial mandate does not operate under similar codes and practices to a professional discipline like social work.

One might ask what right does a group of novice but professionally trained social workers have to question the practice of those outside their organisation who are providing a needed service in a difficult post-disaster situation? A decision to do nothing in this situation poses the risk of putting students with already severely disabling conditions in danger of further injury if untrained volunteers continue to operate complex equipment. Also, doing nothing may mean that students who have already been physically, emotionally and socially traumatised are put in a position of having their right to privacy and confidentiality violated by public exposure on the internet. A decision to act by 'blowing the whistle' on the volunteer group poses a risk for the new social workers in that it may damage the perceived image of the new profession as 'competitive' and 'protecting turf'. While there may be potential for working with the school and community in the future, expressing concerns about the volunteer group's service may limit invitations to do so. In addition, it appears that the new social workers may be acting on their own rather than with the backing of an established professional association that can offer assistance and guidance on such ethical matters.

Ethical dilemmas are often complex and go far beyond simple adherence to a particular code of conduct or practice (rules-based approach). It is our opinion that this situation must be considered with respect to accepted moral or ethical values, but also pragmatism in context.

First, although there may not be a formal code of ethics for social workers in China, other countries that are members of the International Federation of Social Workers include statements in their codes of ethics that highlight the best interests of clients as the primary professional obligation. One could understand this to mean that above all other obligations social workers must ensure that the best interests of vulnerable populations are served. We believe most would agree that this extends beyond the formal 'client-worker' relationship to any groups in society who are in need, and is in keeping with the social justice goals of social work.

Second, social work practice in most countries includes the role of 'advocate' as a legitimate and needed role. Social workers as part of their required practice role are expected to be advocates for their clients and those who are disadvantaged or marginalised.

Although codes of ethics and practice principles for social work in our country, Canada, do not include specific statements about the responsibility for reporting misconduct or inadequate service for other professionals or volunteers, the Australian Association of Social Workers' Code of Ethics is clear in stating that 'social workers will address suspected or confirmed professional misconduct, incompetence, unethical behaviour or negligence by a colleague through appropriate organisational, professional or legal channels' (AASW 2010: 32).

We are of the opinion, therefore, that in this case the social workers have a moral and ethical responsibility to present their concerns about the quality of service being delivered by the volunteer organisation and about the possible abuses of individual rights. However, we also recognise that action should be tempered by a pragmatic and reasoned approach that leads to positive outcomes rather than the mere enforcement of a moral stance.

So, how might these new social workers working in this difficult situation proceed? If inappropriate, unethical or inadequate service is being provided by other professional social workers or other professionals in the same agency, it would be clear that there are appropriate organisational channels to address the concerns. However, again, in this case the situation involves volunteers in a commercial organisation.

We suggest, therefore, that the social workers approach the volunteer group first with their concerns about the rehabilitation service, equipment operation and internet photographs. An offer to work together with them to provide the best service possible to the students might be made. Rather than a 'blowing the whistle' approach on perceived misconduct, we recommend attempts to build bridges with potential partners for better service, and at the same time clearly identifying the areas of concern. This pragmatic approach is balanced as it respects that the volunteer group is providing a needed and valuable service, which the social workers do not wish to be terminated. The goal in this action is not only to advocate for and protect the rights and quality of service, but also to enhance the service.

If the volunteer group is not responsive to the input of the social workers, then we suggest that after weighing the risks, needs and context of the issues, they address their concerns with the principal and the school system. Again, the message conveyed is one that focuses on client service and individual rights as a priority, rather than giving the impression that this is about competition or protection of professional 'turf'.

Recognising that it is important to involve community members in post-disaster management work, there is an opportunity to build capacity at the local level by engaging volunteers. A potential outcome is that the community will be better informed of the role of rehabilitation social work in mainland China in post-disaster contexts.

Reference

Australian Association of Social Workers (2010) *AASW Code of Ethics*, Canberra, ACT: AASW, www.aasw.asn.au/document/item/740, accessed November 2010.

Grant Larson, Ph.D., is Associate Professor, School of Social Work and Human Service, Thompson Rivers University, Kamloops, British Columbia, Canada.
Julie Drolet, Ph.D., is Assistant Professor, School of Social Work and Human Service, Thompson Rivers University, Kamloops, British Columbia, Canada.

Questions for discussion about Case 2.1

1 How helpful do you think clearly formulated ethical codes (like the Australian code mentioned in the second commentary) are to social workers in making decisions in challenging circumstances, such as different political or cultural contexts, disaster situations or countries where social work is newly developing?

2 Using the internet to spread information can have both positive and negative effects. What guidance would you give to the volunteers about how to manage the information on their website in an ethical way?

3 Given the importance in Chinese society of respecting power and hierarchy, and the need to save face, how easy do you think it would be to implement some of the suggestions made by the commentators? What would be *your* advice to the young social workers?

Case study 2.2

Case 2.2: 'When the tables turned': a social work intern's moral dilemma in a Botswana police station

Introduction

This case comes from Botswana. It is about a social work student doing her fieldwork internship at a police station in a city in Botswana. Although many police officers in the country have obtained a diploma or a bachelor's degree in social work from the University of Botswana, they are not deployed as social workers in the police force. Recently, a social work unit was established at the headquarters in the capital city of Gaborone, but this is designed to provide support to police officers themselves rather than to members of the public. Magistrates' courts serve as children's courts in cases of child offending and the magistrate requires a social enquiry report from a social worker, employed by the local authority/council and designated as a probation officer for the purposes of this process. Strictly speaking, there are no probation officers *per se* in Botswana. There are council social workers responsible for liaising with a young person who has broken the law, drawing up a background report, recommending intervention, and providing supervision for a stipulated period after the court case if that is what is decided upon by the magistrate. The young offender might also be sent to the only correctional school of industries in the country for a designated period of time, be sentenced to community service, given corporal punishment, or imprisoned (depending on the nature of the offence and the concomitant circumstances). It has long been a recommendation of the Social Work Department at the University of Botswana and the police service itself that social workers be employed to buttress the efforts of police officers in bringing about positive change in the lives of perpetrators and survivors of crime.

The case

The 17-year-old boy, MTP, sat forlornly and sobbing quietly on a bench in the interview room at the police station. He held his face in his hands. In that posture he looked even younger than his 17 years. Sitting directly opposite him, in a wooden chair, was a young female social work intern who had just completed her third year of studies in the four-year Bachelor of Social Work programme at the University of Botswana. She was clutching a notebook in one hand and a pen in the other. With her face expressionless, she was now, in a quiet voice, saying to the boy for the umpteenth time: 'Both her arms are broken. Doctors say she has internal bleeding. Why did you do this to your mother?'

MTP lifted his head up, with both hands clutching his cheeks. The social work student looked at the boy and could see that he was trembling. 'Would you share with me what happened?' she asked. She had been requested by the police to interview the boy with a view to drawing up a probation officer's report for use at the magistrate's court.

The case against the young boy was essentially that his mother had arrived home late in a drunken stupor, and he had used a pole to beat her up, breaking both arms and a couple of ribs in the process. The police had arrived and, after ensuring that an ambulance had been called and the bleeding mother taken to hospital, they had asked the boy to accompany them to the police station. The boy had spent the entire night in a police cell and the following morning had been interrogated by the police. Later in the day, they requested the social work student to interview the boy and obtain information for a probation officer's report.

'MTP, please share with me what happened', the intern requested. The boy coughed slightly, took a deep breath, and began to speak: 'Eh, if I share the reason with you, do you promise to not tell anyone? You must simply tell people that it was after a misunderstanding involving money.' The intern thought for a moment, scratched her head, and responded: 'It very much depends on the nature of your story, but I cannot promise anything. Tell me about it.'

MTP straightened up, and began to share his story. 'I will start from the beginning, so you can clearly understand the source of my anger.' He then began to explain how he had been born out of wedlock to this, a single mother, and how the mother had shared a single bed with him in their one-roomed rented accommodation. He went on to explain how, when he was very young, his mother would in the middle of the night fondle his sexual organs. When he was a little older his mother would force herself on him on a daily basis. He went on to explain that initially he had totally resented this abuse, but his mother had pleaded with him, misleading him into believing that this was common practice, that most single mothers were 'serviced' by their sons. He explained how, at some point, he had run away from home to a relative's house and only returned when his mother, in confidence, gave him her word that the abuse would stop forthwith. He explained how, as soon as he arrived back home, his mother had pleaded with him to sleep with her 'just this once', and then before he knew it, the abuse resumed in earnest.

'Slowly but surely I began to enjoy it. As I grew older I began to look upon my mother as if she was, say, my wife. I would get enraged when she brought in a boyfriend or arrived back home late without a convincing explanation. When I was 14 or 15 she sensed that I had begun to show signs of aggression and jealousy whenever I "caught" her with a man. I would demand to know who the man was and what his business was. At this point, she tried to stop our "relationship", but by now the tables had been turned. Whereas she had abused me as a young boy all these years, it was now my turn to abuse her. I would demand sex almost on a daily basis. Sometimes she would refuse, saying she was tired, but I would insist. A month ago, I caught her red-handed with a man on our single bed. I told her if I caught her again, I would beat her so badly that she would never walk again, and I meant it. So, yesterday I got back from school early and, when I opened the door using my spare key, I found that a man was lying on top of her, and I just lost my cool.'

At this point the young boy began to sob quietly. The social work intern sat without saying a word – indeed what she was hearing was more than she had bargained for. Her nostrils caught an odour from the boy which she guessed was marijuana. Her mind raced. Should she record this incredible story? Should the boy be turned in for grievous bodily harm? Should she share the story with the police officers? Should she get the police to investigate the drugs issue? The intern simply froze in her chair, not knowing how to proceed.

Commentary 1

GLORIA JACQUES AND RODRECK MUPEDZISWA

There are several ethical/moral issues inherent in this case that pose challenges for professionals working with the two emotionally involved protagonists, mother and son. The complexity of the situation is exacerbated by the fact that it is being addressed by a student intern whose practical experience is limited and whose ability to link theory to practice is still under scrutiny. Furthermore, the probability is that she is being supervised by a police officer who has not had specific training in social work theory and practice. This is one of the ethical issues facing the Department of Social Work at the University of Botswana. Despite the university advocating that police officers with social work qualifications should be employed as social workers in the force, this has not happened. This means that there is no guarantee that interns will be supervised by professional social workers rather than police officers with no specific training in this field.

With regard to the case under discussion, the mother's circumstances would seem, to some extent, to have been dictated by her somewhat convoluted relationship with her young child. She was a single parent, mired in poverty with, probably, few psychosocial support systems. Her situation, in which she shared a single bed with her small son, might have led her to seek comfort through fondling him and (inappropriately) his sexual organs. To her this might have been inextricably related to her circumstances which, in all probability, led her to mistake sex (with the father of her child) for love and caring.

The mother's pleading with her child, when he began to resent the perceived abuse, and justifying it as common practice amongst single mothers, might have been an attempt to rationalise what she no doubt felt might be viewed as unacceptable by society. However, customarily in Botswana it has been the practice for grandparents or elders in the family to touch the sexual organs of young children as an expression of fondness and game playing and thus it is not as foreign as it might appear in the West. Furthermore, she could have known other single mothers in a similar position to herself who acted in the same way with their children and justified the practice to her.

The fact that the boy had run to a relative's home to try to escape the abuse begs the question as to why family members did not investigate the issue and take steps to intervene. Again, culturally influenced factors related to morality might account for this. Firstly, children are meant to be seen and not heard and, secondly, their complaints against their parents would probably not be taken seriously. Thirdly, the aforementioned customary practices involving the touching of sexual organs by elders might have inured family members to such behaviour.

The boy reported that when the abuse resumed following the period when he ran away from home, he gradually began to enjoy it – which could relate to his own feelings of worth and the acceptability of his mother as his historical sexual partner. The child had been socialised to believe that sex between mothers and sons was natural and the comfort arising from an ongoing relationship with someone who showed love to him in every way might have been difficult to refute. The jealousy he felt when his mother had other men in her life appears to have become intolerable as they threatened his somewhat tenuous sense of security and self-worth. She seemingly needed more in the arena of sexual satisfaction than her son could provide and was also possibly obtaining material rewards for her participation with other partners. Furthermore, the mistaken perception of sex as love and acceptance had, in all likelihood, become a lifetime response for her.

The son, possibly infuriated and terrified by the reversal of what he now viewed as a permanent and supportive relationship, believed that he had the right to punish his mother for persuading him against his will initially and then pulling away from him when the tables were turned. This denial of all that they had experienced together appears to have been too much for this confused and insecure teenager. Additionally, his drug-use probably distorted his sense of reality. Although possibly viewed by him as an acceptable coping mechanism, given the trauma of his life, it helped to tip the scales of control and push him over the edge in the belief that he was entitled to react viciously to his mother's behaviour. The pain and confusion of the past 17 years could have blurred his vision and led to an act of extreme violence.

In addressing the case the intern would have to put aside her own prejudices and stereotypical thinking and afford both clients the advantage of being heard and understood as far as possible. Empathic recognition of 'the message behind the message' is essential for professional inter-vention to be effective. Key ethical issues in this case appear to be the woman's distorted view of her relationship with her son; her justification of her behaviour in this regard; and her perceived right to use him for her own purposes and then discard him in favour of other avenues of satisfaction. From the son's perspective his socialisation as a lover and a child would have to be accepted by the student as an important factor in analysing the case. Furthermore, the role of drug-use and the boy's own need for emotional fulfilment (albeit of a sexual nature) is at the forefront of the case. Unravelling these complex factors will prove to be a major challenge for the helper.

At the heart of this problem situation lie the disparate needs of two people inextricably bound by birth and convention. This having been said, both will require assistance in clarifying their own visions of feelings and behaviour acceptable to themselves, significant others and society as a whole. This will be difficult to achieve as the self-serving attitudes of both mother and son tend to obscure the needs of each other. In-depth counselling of both parties will be necessary on an individual and joint basis (if possible) to obtain a rapprochement in the interests of both. This will call for a re-evaluation of themselves and their relationship with each other against a backdrop of ethical sensitivity. The mother will need to restructure her perception of the maternal role in a child's life and the boy should be helped to make sense of factors contributing to his mother's inappropriate behaviour. In the process, both will have to deconstruct their distorted view of parent-child relationships; reconstruct their vision of appropriate behaviour; and, if possible, reconstruct their relationship with one another. Depending on the extent of the damage it might be possible to establish a foundation for mutual respect. In the event that this is impossible, then coming to terms with the past and charting a future separate from each other but involving significant others in a more conducive manner might be the only realistic conclusion.

Gloria Jacques is Senior Lecturer, Department of Social Work, University of Botswana.

Rodreck Mupedziswa is Associate Professor and Head, Department of Social Work, University of Botswana.

Commentary 2

PETA-ANNE BAKER

So many alarm bells go off in my head as I read this case. From a social work educator perspective one of my first questions is: 'Where is this student's supervisor?' No undergraduate student should have to deal with a case like this on her own. I suspect, however, that if the situation in Botswana is like that in Jamaica, her supervisor is so happy that there is an extra pair of hands to share some of the workload that s/he may not have been careful about making sure the intern would be able to handle any matters that came her way and would know how to recognise when she was getting in over her head.

In Jamaica there would actually only be one decision that could be taken, since the Child Care and Protection Act (2004)[3] requires the mandatory reporting of all cases of child abuse. In fact, while all members of society are required to make reports of even suspected abuse or neglect, members of 'prescribed' groups, such as social work, are under an even greater obligation and face severe penalties for failing to do so.

A young student would certainly need help not only in understanding the law, which she would have studied in the classroom setting, but also in dealing with the feelings which MTP's account would evoke. Most importantly in the immediate situation, she would need help in clarifying her role: is she there to help the police make their case, or is she really an agent of the court (which would be the case if she were a probation officer)? Her initial words seem to suggest that she starts out wearing her agent of social control hat: 'Both her arms are broken, why did you do this to your mother?' But as MTP's own unhappiness and possibly fear become more apparent, we can see that our intern is probably struggling with feelings of sympathy and a desire to help. Does she handle well the issue of MTP's request for confidentiality (indeed his request that she lie)? Not really, but under the circumstances this is probably understandable.

Many of us as social workers are not comfortable with our contradictory roles: agents of social control as well as social change. In any event, since most social workers in developing countries are employed by the state, it is the social control function that is often the most prominent. Sometimes we try to downplay that role, as the intern does when she provides a less than definitive response to MTP's request not only to keep what he is about to tell her in confidence, but actually to lie about it. Not many of us get into the profession because we want to ensure that people fit into society's norms. Indeed, many see social work as a means of defending the rights of the poor and the vulnerable, so one can readily see that the intern would feel that she is confronted with a choice between her obligation to society and her obligation to the young person (child in the legal sense of the term) in front of her.

It also seems that MTP may not be clear about why the intern is interviewing him. The case does not indicate whether he was provided with an explanation of why she was there. Again, sometimes in the heat of the moment, we do not provide a clear explanation of what our role is and what the client can expect from us. Indeed, in the context of the foregoing discussion about social work's social control function, one might be tempted to wonder who the client is in this situation: MTP or the police (who want a report)?

3 http://www.cda.gov.jm/child_care_protection_act.php

As if the intern has not been sufficiently challenged, she smells what she thinks might be marijuana. This is possibly where the student's youthfulness becomes most apparent since if MTP has spent the night in jail then it was just as possible that the smell came from his association with others as from his own usage. How would he have obtained it if he has been in custody? My own instinct based very much on Jamaican attitudes to this drug would be to ignore this additional factor; a government appointed commission has actually recommended decriminalisation of possession of small amounts.

Finally, I am concerned about the expectation that a recommendation could be made to the court on the basis of a single interview with an obviously disturbed young person, who has just himself endured and participated in another series of traumatising events. Truth be told, no real dilemma exists, although an inexperienced intern may think otherwise. The course of action in the Jamaican context, at least, would be clear. The student needs to provide her young client (and the police officers) with a brief explanation of what her next steps will be, immediately contact her supervisor, and provide a report on what she has learned so that they can seek to secure appropriate psychological and legal assistance for their young client. Regrettably, at least in the Jamaican context, there is no guarantee that he would speedily receive either, which might call forth the intern's need to learn what it is to play another important professional role, that of advocate.

Dr Peta-Anne Baker is Coordinator of the Social Work Programme at the University of the West Indies, Mona Campus in Jamaica. She teaches the professional ethics course in the school's graduate programme.

Questions for discussion about Case 2.2

1 In your opinion, is it justifiable that the police should ask a social work student to interview the boy in order to obtain information about the case, especially if there is no supervision available from a social worker?
2 Taking the social and cultural background into consideration, what is your view about the boy's account of his sexual relationship with his mother? How would an incestuous relationship like this be regarded in your own society?
3 What would you advise the social work student to do in this situation?

Case 2.3: When is it right to accept a gift? A Lithuanian social work student's dilemma

Introduction

This case is written by a social work academic in Lithuania. The studies of social work are organised at the university in the centre of Lithuania, a former republic of the Soviet Union. The development of the social work profession in Lithuania began in 1992, after the collapse of the Soviet Union. When Lithuania became a politically independent state and responsible for its own borders, it became a transition country for refugees to the European Union (EU) from other former Soviet Union republics and Asian countries. With the support of other EU countries, an agreement was made to organise a camp for refugees and a reception centre for asylum seekers. Further integration of the asylum seekers is organised through an NGO (non-governmental organisation) support centre for the integration of refugees. Social work students are placed in this NGO for their fieldwork placements. This particular case relates to refugees from Chechenia, a federal republic of Russia, which experienced intense battles in the 1990s in struggles for independence, with sporadic fighting still continuing in some areas.

The case

Lina was a student in the fourth year of her baccalaureate, studying social work. I was her teacher of ethics in social work. During her field placement she was working at the special programme for families with children from Chechenia. There was no course in the social work educational programmes about immigrants, refugees, or other cultures in Lithuania. The course about ethics in social work was taught after the term in which the fieldwork placement occurred. Lina came to me and presented this case as a situation about which she was still thinking. Lina worked with two families with children during one term for two days per week. She had a tutor from the university, who helped her to learn from practice, and a mentor at this NGO. During the practice she worked very successfully with one family. She helped this family to organise support for their child at school, helped to find a job for the father, and helped the family to get a permanent social home (flat) in the city. She worked as a consultant and as an advocate for each of the family members, and for the family as a whole. At the closing of the case, at the meeting with all family members, the mother gave her a silver bracelet as a gift for her very significant support to their family. Lina felt confused in this situation. As Lina told me, she tried not to accept this gift, but the mother insisted that she should accept, and so she did. But still she had a question: Was she right to do this?

Her reasons for accepting this gift were that she did not want to outrage the mother and she did not know the traditions and culture of the Chechenians. She did not discuss this issue with her tutor during the practice. We analysed this case in the classroom and the group decided that Lina was right to accept this gift. But some questions were raised, including: Is it enough to discuss this case after the fieldwork practice? Is the group decision the right way to solve the situation? What next steps should be taken to avoid similar questions arising for other students working in multicultural areas?

Commentary 1

NINO ZGANEC

The case of the social work student from Lithuania opens a range of important questions that face social workers all around the world when they work with their clients in social work practice. I will try in my commentary to reflect some of these questions and will also discuss some elements of this situation as they may appear in other cultural contexts, such as Croatia, where I am based.

Social workers who are involved in the process of helping, whether on a paid or voluntary basis, whether as part of their student practice or as professional work 'need to acknowledge that they are accountable for their actions to the users of their services, the people they work with, their colleagues, their employers, the professional association and to the law, and that these accountabilities may conflict' (IFSW and IASSW 2004). This accountability in professional practice is challenged very often by specific circumstances that occur in the process of helping and that may arise from cultural specificity, as in this case.

The question of cultural specificity places demands on social workers to recognise diversity, as the IFSW and IASSW (2004) statement on ethics in social work says: 'Social workers should recognise and respect the ethnic and cultural diversity of the societies in which they practise, taking account of individual, family, group and community differences.' The student of social work in Lithuania apparently was successful in her work with the family, but according to her own judgement she was not well enough informed about the traditions and culture of the Chechenians. These kinds of situations can pose serious problems for social workers and can open some ethical dilemmas, as in this case. But a question that we may also ask is: How would the student react if she was informed about the culture and tradition of the Chechenians? I guess that a stable relationship of trust and respect was established between the student and family members, which resulted in the wish of the family to thank the person who significantly improved their life. The gift item – in this case a silver bracelet – apparently is in accordance with the values cherished by the Chechenian family.

One question we can ask is whether the process of respecting ethnic and cultural diversity assumes a deviation from the professional values of social workers? The answer is certainly 'no'. But, at the same time, one can ask a second question: whether the acceptance of the silver bracelet as a gift and thanks for the support to the family amounts to a deviation from the professional values of social workers? In answering this second question we need to know more about the professional values of social work in a particular society (in this case Lithuania). In other words, we should always consider cultural specificity and the context in which social work takes place. Indeed, we should consider not just cultural specificity but also legal and ethical regulations and norms. For instance, is the acceptance of this kind of gift allowed by law? Is this situation prescribed by the ethical code of the national professional organisation? And finally, is this kind of behaviour, generally speaking, regarded as ethical in the society?

The situation in my native country, Croatia, shows that in previous decades it was common to give gifts to people in professional positions as a symbol of gratitude. At the time this led to the situation where some of the professions almost came into disrepute because they were accused of bribery and corruption. The important question to consider here is where is the dividing line between the culturally acceptable receipt of gifts and the receipt of gifts that over time becomes a requirement for the provision of quality services? We can say that the issue of professionalism, and especially the question of professional boundaries between professionals and clients, is more important than ever. This does not mean not accepting cultural diversity; rather, it means respecting the profession on behalf of which a service is provided. The acceptance of gifts can be at the same time an insult for the client whom I help, as well as an insult for me as a social worker. If the client insists on giving a gift this can represent a disregard of my profession and the professional work that I have done. When we interpret too widely the principle of acceptance or understanding of cultural diversity this can lead to the dismantling of the professional boundaries between social workers and clients.

We can consider this issue within the framework of ethical absolutism or ethical relativism. Consistent and thorough acceptance of cultural diversity and specificity arises from a relativist position, which entails that the decision is made on the basis of taking into account the particular circumstances and contexts in which the work is taking place. The absolutist (deontological) position requires that principles of what counts as acceptable and unacceptable behaviour from social workers are defined in advance and are applicable in all circumstances. This latter position, of course, does not reject the giving of respect to cultural diversity, but it is led by this diversity when the ethical principles and rules are made, and requires that it should be respected by both the social worker and the client. The normal prerequisite for this to work well is that both social workers and clients are familiar with the ethical rules that apply in the process of professional helping.

We can see from this case how important it is in social work for professional workers to clarify their roles and boundaries at the start of any professional helping relationship, and how important it is to clarify mutual rights and duties, possibilities and expectations. The dangers of failing to clarify adequately the ground rules operating in professional helping are pervasive and lurk around every corner of the work. Even after the work is finished, they can return like a boomerang bringing us into a situation in which we feel confusion, hurt, lack of success or at least we have a serious ethical dilemma.

Reference

International Federation of Social Workers and International Association of Schools of Social Work (2004) *Ethics in Social Work, Statement of Principles*, www.ifsw.org, accessed October 2010.

Nino Zganec is Associate Professor at the Study Centre of Social Work in the Faculty of Law at the University of Zagreb, Croatia.

Commentary 2

HOWARD SERCOMBE

On the face of it, the giving of a gift, and its acceptance, is entirely appropriate within the ethics of normal human relationships. Helping someone in trouble if they need it, without going too much out of your way – what Reiman (1990) calls 'easy rescue' – is an ethical obligation in human relationships. Lina's effort goes beyond this general duty to help. It is not surprising that the family feels grateful; in such circumstances, gratitude to the person who has helped is also a moral obligation. A gift is a common and appropriate way to express that gratitude, and to offer it is a tangible and, in this case, enduring symbol of the relationship. There are a number of caveats, however, which have together led to a tradition in social work and other professions of not accepting gifts from clients.

First, it is common for interactions to become distorted by the belief that an act of grace leaves one indebted. We live in an individualistic society, in which there seems to be a great fear of commitment or obligation to others. The gift, then, is not a symbol of gratitude, but is about the payment of the debt and any implication that one might be obliged to return help if called upon to do so. The encounter is then moved into an exchange, even a commercial transaction, in which the bracelet is payment for work done. The gift, if it is overly generous, could even be intended to create a reverse debt, which could be called on at some future time. Conversely, rejection of the gift could be understood as a manipulative desire on Lina's part to maintain the debt, so that it could be called in at a time and place of Lina's choosing. The constitution of the relationship as contractual, of symmetrical or commercial exchange, is a distortion of the professional relationship (Koehn 1994).

This brings us to the next point. This is not an ordinary human relationship. It is a professional relationship, specifically, a social work relationship. Lina's work is not an act of grace, even though it might feel like one. While she is engaging and skilful in the way that she does her work, that is her duty, and to do less would be to fall short of her duty. Therefore gratitude, in the measure that is evident in the giving of the bracelet, is not called for. We may thank people for doing what they are supposed to do, but this is a matter of courtesy, rather than obligation. There is a problem if a culture of expectation of a gift develops, or worse, that delivering a service becomes contingent on a gift being offered. That would be corruption.

Third, the sense of gratitude indicates that the relationship has been allowed to be constructed as an exchange in which Lina is helping this family to get their lives together; an enterprise in which she is successful. This construction is carried in the case description: Lina is the active party, the family is passive. This is not our preferred understanding of social work practice, where ideally it is the client who does the work. We (social workers) facilitate, we help, but we are catalytic in the process, not determinant. If this approach were followed, we might imagine rewriting the case description as follows:

> During the practice, one family especially took Lina on. The family worked hard to show her what they needed and how to work collaboratively with them. By using her cultural capital and status, the family was able to organise support for their child at school, the father found a job, and the family successfully found and moved into a permanent social home (flat) in the city. Each of the family members took the time and the risk to bring Lina into their confidence, to educate her sufficiently regarding their very different social and cultural experience, and to trust her to speak on their behalf.

This alternative construction of the case would place Lina in less of a helping role, and hence less inclined to regard gratitude as a legitimate response. It might also guard against the danger of transference, which is especially real in this situation. Transference is when a client projects onto a professional 'feelings that are really to do with their own process and their own journey' (Sercombe 2010: 102). Clearly, the relationship between Lina and this family has been transformative for the family and probably also for Lina. Because Lina is 'the professional', and because she is the new term in the equation of their lives, it is easy for the family to think that she is wonderful and that she has brought about all these good things, which they never would have been able to do: that she has saved them. This is very flattering, and it would be tempting for Lina to believe this too, though there are no indications that she does. But it would be just as appropriate for Lina to buy each member of the family presents for allowing her into their lives and allowing her, as a student, to learn the things that they have taught her.

If this was an ordinary relationship, if Lina was a neighbour, the giving of a gift like this would be entirely appropriate. The fact that it is not appropriate here points to the fact that this is a very different kind of relationship to being a neighbour, even though that is what it might feel like. The family may have no experience of this kind of professional relationship, and the only templates that they might have for understanding how the relationship works might be family or neighbour templates. It can be really difficult to establish a professional social work relationship on the right kind of footing, and the silver bracelet seems to indicate that Lina might not have successfully done that as thoroughly and cleanly as we might hope. That being the case, it is now difficult to refuse the gift without seeming churlish. The relationship being what the relationship is, the understanding being what the understanding is, it was right for Lina to accept the bracelet.

However, this silver bracelet represents an opportunity for Lina to renegotiate the relationship. The case description does not make it clear whether Lina still has access to the family, but I can imagine her going back and saying: 'I've thought about this, and I don't think this bracelet belongs to me. You have all worked hard, with lots of courage. I want to give this back to you as a symbol of what you have achieved.'

The case description asks a number of questions about how this problem was treated. To deal with the last question first, in order to prevent this happening again, Lina and her colleagues need a firm grounding in the nature of the professional relationship, particularly the social work relationship: what is special about it, and what rewards each party can legitimately expect from the relationship. If they are clean and clear in their practice (which does not exclude being kind, friendly or caring) then clients like the Chechenian family cannot but take up the responsive role.

In terms of the way that the episode was treated, the offering of the gift, and its acceptance, immediately represented an ethical dilemma, which Lina knew and felt. Immediately, she should have discussed this with her supervisor or tutor; that she did not do this means that Lina needs to think about her own responsibility in terms of confronting this boundary violation. In the moment, I think accepting the bracelet was reasonable, as long as it was not too expensive (if it was expensive it has to go back as soon as possible). A mistake was made, and we usually discover that an ethical line has been crossed after we have crossed it and, to mix metaphors, we hear the ice cracking. The point then is to fix it if we can, and if we cannot, to learn what we can both about the ethics of it and about ourselves as the person who got into that position (Buber 1965). Retrospective analysis (we would call it reflective practice) is not only useful in this journey, it is critical.

Groups or panels of our peers are a useful way to work this through: not only to guard against our tendency for rationalisation and self-deception but also to spread the conversation wider so that others have access to our learning without having to make the mistake themselves. The only caution, particularly in a profession where empathy is the central essential attribute, is the tendency in such groups to excuse each other, especially in the face of discomfort. If we are not clean and clear enough, we endorse and reinforce bad practice, and we do not learn the things we need to learn.

References

Buber, M. (1965) 'Guilt and guilt feelings' in M. Buber (ed.) *The Knowledge of Man*, New York: Harper and Row.

Koehn, D. (1994) *The Ground of Professional Ethics*, London: Routledge.

Reiman, J. (1990) *Justice and Modern Moral Philosophy*, New Haven: Yale University Press.

Sercombe, H. (2010) *Youth Work Ethics*, London: Sage.

Howard Sercombe is Professor of Community Education at the University of Strathclyde, Glasgow, Scotland.

Questions for discussion about Case 2.3

1   Are there occasions when you think it might be ethically acceptable in social work to accept gifts from service users?
2   How is it possible to distinguish professional and personal aspects of a relationship between a social worker and a service user? How helpful are ethical codes and guidelines in situations like this?
3   In this case, was it the responsibility of the student or the supervisor to decide whether to accept the gift?

Case study 2.4

Case 2.4: 'Why should I have to reveal anything about my personal life?' A dilemma for a lesbian student in Britain

Introduction

This case is from a British social work student undertaking fieldwork practice in a residential children's home. The case focuses on the question of whether the student, who identifies herself as lesbian, should reveal this to her colleagues in the residential home. In Britain, lesbianism is a recognised sexual identity – for example, civil partnerships between same-sex couples are now recognised in law. However, in society generally there is still widespread discrimination against lesbians.

The case

Anna was a young female student (aged 20) in her second year of study on a Bachelor's programme in social work at a British university. She was undertaking her first fieldwork practice placement, which lasted 80 days, as a social care worker in a small residential home for young people with behavioural problems. The residential home was privately run, comprising six single rooms. It accommodated children and young people on full care orders, interim care orders and accommodation orders under the Children Act 1989, with the aim of maintaining and promoting the young people's health and well-being and helping them to gain a positive future as adults. The young people were 15 and 16 years old. The staff included a manager, deputy manager, five care workers and two 'bank' (temporary) workers. The placement involved Anna working shifts during the daytime, evenings and weekends. Another older female student in her third year of study from a neighbouring university was also on placement at the residential home at the same time as Anna.

Anna was allocated as a key worker for a troubled boy, with whom she developed a good relationship over a period of several weeks. The boy was 15 years old, hence not much younger than Anna. She was pleased that he was responding to her and making good progress in the home and at school. She worked hard at maintaining the relationship in a professional way, but became aware that he was attracted to her. She discussed this with her supervisor, but was shocked to learn that the staff felt that she was acting unprofessionally and was developing much too close a relationship with the boy. They did not realise she was a lesbian, and were assuming that she was developing some kind of sexual relationship with him. She was put under further pressure when the other student on placement at the home also made the same assumption and reported her relationship with the boy to the staff. Anna was very reluctant to reveal the fact that she was a lesbian, but feared that her own student placement was in jeopardy as well as the relationship with and the progress of the service user – from whom she was being advised to withdraw. She raised the question: 'Why should I have to reveal anything about my personal life?'

Commentary 1

NICKI WARD

In providing a commentary that focuses on the ethical dimensions of this case study, I will begin with Anna's question: 'Why should I have to reveal anything about my personal life?' and will consider whether Anna's sexuality is relevant in the context of her practice as a social work student. I will outline three different sets of reasons that might be used to justify disclosure of her sexuality.

1 *Disclosure as protection* – on the face of it, Anna's reasons for considering disclosing her sexuality are defensive, driven by a belief that doing so will defuse and undermine the assumptions being made against her. In this context it might be argued that she should not have to reveal anything about her personal life. Doing so may resolve the immediacy of the situation for her, in as much as her colleagues may stop making assumptions about her being sexually predatory and wanting to develop an inappropriate intimate relationship with a young man. However, it will not address what I see to be the under-lying ethical issue here: the impact of the heterosexist and hetero-normative values of Anna's colleagues. The critique of Anna's practice would seem to be more reflective of their values and heteronormative assumptions than of Anna's behaviour. In this sense, Anna's sexuality is irrelevant as these values and beliefs still need to be explored and challenged. Given Anna's role as a student social worker, then the ethical responsibility could be seen to belong to Anna's supervisor.

2 *Disclosure as defusion* – the second reason Anna might consider disclosing is to try to defuse the situation further with the young man for whom she is key worker, whom we know is becoming attracted to her. However, irrespective of Anna's sexuality, there is a need for Anna and the young man to be able to develop and maintain a professional and platonic relationship. Whilst disclosure may make it clear to the young man that Anna is not attracted to him, it will not necessarily stop him being attracted to her and could also inadvertently give him the message that if she were not a lesbian 'things would be different'. The important issue here, however, is to enable this young man to understand the boundaries, helping him to gain a clearer understanding of how to develop positive relationships with both men and women in a range of different situations. Given that the aims of the residential home are to maintain and promote

young people's health and well-being and to help them gain a positive future as adults, this might seem a more ethical and value-based response.

The discussion above suggests that the fact that Anna is a lesbian is irrelevant and that she should not have to reveal anything about her personal life for reasons of protecting herself or defusing the situation with the young man. However, in the context of *practising* social work ethics we might view this differently. The problem with ethics often is that we are trying to make a decision based on a cognitive assessment of the situation. This gives the impression that what we are doing is making a simple decision based on universal moral principles, objectively weighing the 'pros and cons'. But where these situations involve personal identity and beliefs, as they so often do, they are not rational cognitive decisions and their impact is felt not only by us, but also by others within the relationship. Ethical decision-making, therefore, needs to be contextual and relational. Anna's decision has to be taken in the context of the impact it will have on her, but also the impact it will have on others within her wider social network. This leads to a third set of reasons for disclosure, namely, as challenge.

3   *Disclosure as challenge* – central to social work values and ethics are notions that social workers should work anti-oppressively, promoting inclusion and challenging discrimination. Issues of heteronormativity and heterosexism are often hidden; because society is dominated by heterosexuality it becomes easy to assume that this is how life is for everyone. Being open about your sexuality can help to challenge these assumptions and to make people more aware of their behaviour and how it might impact on those who do not identify as heterosexual. In this sense, Anna coming out as a lesbian may serve as a catalyst for encouraging her colleagues to reflect on their own values and assumptions about sexuality and consider how this might impact on others around her. Similarly, disclosing her sexuality to the young man with whom she works, and to other young people within the home, could also provide a catalyst for the young people, contributing to the establishment's wider aims around well-being and positive futures and providing the positive lesbian role models that are so often missing from young people's lives.

In considering the response to her question: 'Why should I have to reveal anything about my personal life?' Anna needs to decide how she balances her personal rights (either to privacy, or to respect for her life and who she is) with her responsibilities (to the service user with whom she is working, to the social work profession and, potentially, to the wider lesbian, gay and bisexual community). I believe that the right thing to do in this situation is to disclose, not in order to defend herself, but to challenge discriminatory practice and promote inclusion. But this can only be done in a context in which Anna feels safe and supported.

Nicki Ward is Lecturer in Social Work, School of Social Policy, University of Birmingham, UK.

Commentary 2

JOAN C. TRONTO

Anna's reluctance to 'reveal something personal' raises two important ethical questions about how to maintain a boundary between one's private and professional life. First: how does one keep a proper distance between one's personal and professional life? Second: should our answer to this question change for gays and lesbians?

What is the proper distance between personal and professional life?

Being 'ethical' always happens in a context. Professionals need to keep a proper professional distance from clients. But what is 'proper'? Acting ethically in a professional setting is not only about a person's private feelings about what is proper, but also about professional standards and shared understandings about acting rightly. As a professional, Anna assumes certain professional responsibilities. Many thinkers who make 'responsibility' central to their accounts of morality emphasise that, at its root, responsibility is linked to 'response,' that is, to an existing relationship. In this case, as in most cases, the relationships that shape their responsibilities are various.

Professionals are almost always in relationships of *asymmetric power* with their clients. As a result, they need to be wary of ways in which their position might permit them to impose harm upon, or have undue influence over, clients. One of the reasons that some colleges and universities in the United States, for example, have banned all intimate relationships between faculty and students is because of the danger that personal relationships blur attraction and power in ways that might make judgement about the situation impossible. Sexual relationships are especially difficult to sort out; it is one reason why all forms of sexual harassment are forbidden.

Given that clients of social workers have needs for the workers' care, an imbalance of power is always present. If it cannot be eliminated, is there a way to remove the moral danger that professionals will take advantage of their charges from such relationships? There is – through a process of supervision and peer review so that the other workers can raise questions about the worker's relationship to the client on the client's behalf.

Anna also has relationships with, and responsibilities to, the other social workers. Some of these relationships are among equals, others are also hierarchical. The responsibilities to co-workers and to one's supervisors, or to those one supervises, are also different because they entail different levels of power. In this case, one disturbing feature is that the other student had spoken to the supervisor but not to Anna herself. Why not? In all relationships of caring, including those within a professional organisation, there is a danger of paternalism, i.e., that the values of the more powerful actors (social worker or supervisor), rather than the actual needs of the one who is receiving the care, will define the caring needs. Is Anna's conduct actually wrong, or are her co-workers overly sensitive to this issue? Whose judgement is influencing the outcome of this case? Is the supervisor relying too much upon the others' views?

Anna's biggest problem here was not that she was engaged in a sexual relationship with the client, she was not. The problem was that others perceived her relationship with the client to have become a sexual one. Is this Anna's problem? In part it is not; clearly, others had leaped to an inaccurate conclusion. In part, though, Anna needs to think much more about her multiple responsibilities and how her conduct appears to others: both to the client and to the other professionals in this setting.

Are there specific issues for gays and lesbians?

Since Anna's defence against the charge that she was improperly close to the boy was that she was a lesbian, must she disclose that fact? If Anna does not wish her own sexuality to become an issue, then she must avoid a situation in which it becomes an issue. But being a lesbian does not protect her from a situation in which a young male client is sexually attracted to her. So even if she had disclosed her sexual identity to her supervisor and co-workers, the issue of the client's attraction would still arise. So, on one level, she does not need to 'come out' to solve this problem, and coming out does not solve it.

But perhaps Anna should 'come out' at work nonetheless. Why? Sexual identity is a particular case. Unlike many other stigmatised identities, for example, gender, race, language, there is no way for others to know that one is gay/lesbian unless one discloses it. Gays and lesbians can, and often do, 'pass' for 'normal' in most settings, thereby sparing themselves the harm of overt discrimination. There are other costs of leading a life in hiding, of course, such as feeling as if one is living a lie. And gays and lesbians frequently argue that one reason to end discrimination is because this burden of being less than completely truthful is a serious moral cost for gays and lesbians to bear.

Anna might want to consider her membership of a community that is not well regarded as another responsibility. Although being a lesbian is still stigmatised in the UK, and, indeed, even criminal in other places in the world, is it better to hide one's identity or to make it public? Research shows that one of the best indicators of increasing tolerance for gays and lesbians is that people who say that they know a gay or lesbian person are more likely to be tolerant of gays and lesbians. Coming out, then, increases tolerance. Anna does not have a strict responsibility to come out in order to make life easier for other gays and lesbians. But if she considers herself not only as an individual but as a member of this somewhat invisible and disliked community, then maybe she will see that coming out is not only about revealing something personal.

Must Anna disclose something personal? Perhaps not. But if she wishes to avoid the appearance of inappropriate actions, then she needs to consider not only her own perspective but the perspectives of her clients, co-workers, and agency as well. She needs to realise that professional distance is often necessary, not only to protect social workers but also to protect clients.

Joan C. Tronto is Professor of Political Science at the University of Minnesota, USA. She is the author of *Moral Boundaries: A Political Argument for an Ethic of Care* (1993) and continues to write about ethics and politics from a care perspective. She is also a lesbian who has been 'out' for more than 30 years.

Questions for discussion about Case 2.4

1 The challenge of building a close relationship with a service user and at the same time keeping a professional distance is a well-known ethical issue for professional workers. What similar

experiences have you had in struggling to get the right balance of closeness and distance? Why do you think it is such a difficult issue for social workers?

2 Do you see the student's sexual identity as the main issue in this case? Explain the reasons for your answer.

3 If the student in this case came to you for advice about what to do, what would you say and why? What would you do if you were the student in this case?

<table>
<tr><td>3</td><td># Respecting rights</td></tr>
</table>

Introduction

LINDA BRISKMAN AND MARÍA JESÚS ÚRIZ PEMÁN

Human rights and social work

In this introduction we will focus on human rights in the context of social work practice. A human rights discourse has gained prominence and widespread recognition over the last half century, although defined in various ways. A simple way to describe human rights is as universal entitlements that belong to all human beings in respect of being human and regardless of such factors as national origin, race, culture, age or gender (Ife 2001). It is a powerful discourse, which seeks to overcome divisiveness and sectarianism and unite people from all walks of life through asserting human values and the universality of humanity (ibid.).

Human rights have been defined and understood in different ways throughout history, shifting and changing in response to changes in society and different social movements. Over time, perceptions of human rights have changed to encompass changes in the demographic make-up of societies. However, there are still individuals and groups of people at the margins of societies whose rights are not fully protected or realised (Black 2008).

For social work there are arguably challenges facing the incorporation of a human rights perspective into education, policy and practice. One is the view that the concept of human rights is a legal concept alone and the domain of lawyers, with its primary focus on international and domestic law. To ensure a broader and more inclusive understanding of human rights, social workers can widen the approach from the legal sphere through reconceptualising human rights frameworks to include the moral, political, policy and practice spheres of knowledge.

A second tension is moving social work from a discourse that privileges needs, care and service provision over rights. Human services delivery is often framed within welfarist and needs-based paradigms (Briskman 2007a), resulting in potential for an apparent clash of paradigms. Rioux and Zubrow (2001) in their work on disability provide some leads for reframing the approach to dealing with vulnerable people, which in the case of disability rights requires moving from a pathologising or bio-medical lens to a reformulation of economic, social and political policy. This is not always an easy quest as human service organisations can be resistant to change (Briskman 2007b), particularly in a global climate where neo-liberalism prevails. One way of overcoming the tensions is to see social work as contributing to the development of a 'rights culture', wherein understandings of rights go beyond the legal frameworks of protection and enforcement and where concepts of rights transcend disciplines and become integrated in society at many levels. In this framework human rights are understood not as a panacea for all injustices but as a discursive and analytical tool to foster societal change (Fiske and Briskman 2008).

A human rights approach is powerful for transformational social work. Such a framework can provide social workers with a moral basis for their practice (Ife 2001). How to incorporate human rights in societies has occupied social workers, educators, philosophers, lawyers and politicians for a very long time (Reichert 2003). Human rights are implicitly at the heart of social work and their most overt application is enshrinement in both international and national codes of ethics. Despite the quest by some academics and practitioners to see social work positioned as a human rights profession there are a number of points of contention. These include the question of rights versus responsibilities and the issue of whether social work should adopt a 'universalist' or 'cultural relativist' approach to human rights, which will be discussed more fully later. From a practitioner perspective, the difficulty of applying human rights tenets to practice remains vexed as revealed in the cases in this chapter.

The International Federation of Social Workers (IFSW) has developed a policy on social work and human rights and, together with the International Association of Schools of Social Work (IASSW), has formulated a definition of social work that states explicitly that human rights are fundamental to social work. In a number of countries, a commitment to human rights in social work is included in national social work codes of ethics. The IFSW and IASSW (2004) document on *Ethics in Social Work: Statement of Principles* brings to the forefront human rights and human dignity:

> Social work is based on respect for the inherent worth and dignity of all people and the rights that follow from this. Social workers should uphold and defend each person's physical, psychological, emotional and spiritual integrity and well-being.
>
> (IFSW and IASSW 2004: para. 4.1)

Social work is a profession that is laden with uncertainties and contradictions. It often has trouble situating itself in relation to more dominant professions such as law, medicine and psychiatry, and in some settings it struggles with identity and role and a professional power imbalance – an aspect that is particularly evident in Case 3.1 about a social worker in a psychiatric hospital. Furthermore, social work is sometimes seen in a dichotomous way, divided between 'conservative' and 'progressive' approaches. Perhaps unfairly, those working at the micro-level of direct social work practice may be accused of perpetuating unjust systems and not working towards social justice and social change. Dominelli (1998) suggests that the role and purpose of social work has been contested since its inception, with three approaches evident: therapeutic helping; maintenance; and emancipation. Arguably, however, at whatever level of practice and in whatever setting, social work can make a contribution to emancipatory practice that overturns human rights violations, even through small steps as the cases in this chapter illustrate.

Unlike the participants in these cases, who exercise courage by admitting they are stumped by human rights contemplations, it is perhaps regrettable that there are not more robust endeavours to enshrine human rights practice within the social work profession. One of the stumbling blocks is social work education itself, with educators frequently lamenting the crowded curriculum and competition between competing paradigms that can lead to human rights avoidance. However, through contact with groups who struggle to achieve their human rights, social workers will become aware of human rights directives at a number of levels. For example, some groups may struggle to have their civil and political rights (also known as first generation rights) recognised, while others lack the amenities for the realisation of their economic, social and cultural rights (second generation rights). Still others have problems with the achievement of collective rights (third generation rights). Further discussion on the three generations of rights can be found in Ife (2008).

When considering the cases in this chapter, we need to recognise that human rights approaches to social work cohere with much social work theorising. The vision of human rights builds on other emancipatory paradigms, such as anti-racism, feminism, critical postmodernism and post-colonialism. Nonetheless, there are contradictions for social workers in the actual implementation of the theoretical constructs – including the complexities of balancing personal, professional and political issues and operating within constrained environments (Cemlyn 2008). In most of the cases in this chapter the practitioners are employed by social service organisations that can limit their own autonomy as well as that of the people whose interests they purport to represent.

Contested ground

It is important for social workers to be cognisant of the Universal Declaration of Human Rights (United Nations 1948), which was a great achievement for all of humankind. What it advocates is that there are common principles of humanity that apply to everyone, regardless of class, gender, ethnicity, age, ability and religion. As Ife (2008) notes, the UDHR is an inspirational document that has been used in many ways to further many important causes for humanity.

Nonetheless social workers should recognise the critiques of the content of codified international standards, including the UDHR, particularly the criticism of cultural imperialism. This essentially revolves around the 'universal' construction that argues that human rights should be adopted by all peoples and cultures, and the 'cultural relativist' approach that contends that we need to contest the position of universal 'moral truths' which may not be applicable to non-Western cultures (Nipperess and Briskman 2009). Accusations are sometimes levelled at Western constructs of human rights; and human services practitioners in non-Western settings are generally more adept at negotiating the balance between the universal and the culturally specific. This is particularly evident in Case 3.3 where a Dutch student working in Vietnam is displaced from practice norms that are part of Western social work practice. Such practice dilemmas may not just occur away from the social worker's home country, but can also create the need to wrestle with issues of cultural diversity within a framework that combines multicultural and human rights perspectives. The ability to walk in another's shoes should perhaps be a core human rights tenet for social workers.

In order to respond to ethical practice dilemmas social workers need to be up to date with the human rights debates about 'universalism' and 'cultural relativism'. Elizabeth Reichert (2003) points out the tensions. In terms of universality, she highlights the position that every individual has a claim to enjoy human rights. These rights, she says, include, for example, adequate health care and nutrition for all. However, she points out that not all human rights are as clear-cut, as the examples in this chapter indicate. The notion of universality may clash with particular cultures, laws, policies, morals and regimes that fail to recognise the human rights in question. She asks what should prevail – the cultural or religious norm or the human right. This raises questions such as the following, which social workers must consider in their human rights judgements and which can be applied to the cases in this chapter (ibid.):

- Who defines a human right?
- Who benefits from the definition?
- Who loses from the definition?
- Whose voices are being heard in enforcing human rights?
- Who defines culture?
- Does one government have the right to tell another government that its policies violate a human right?

Nipperess and Briskman (2009) respond to some of the critiques of both positions, pointing out that although modern Western thinkers have clearly influenced much of the thinking on human rights, this does not mean that the idea of human rights is not relevant to the rest of the world. Notions of human rights have, in fact, been discussed for millennia and cultures other than those in the West have contributed to the dialogue. There is hence a distinction to be made between the term 'human rights' and the concept of human rights, in that the term may be perceived as a modernist entity, whereas the idea of human rights and shared humanity is not a product of modernity. They also point out the criticisms of the cultural relativist position that suggest that human rights violations may thrive in the name of culture. Relativists have been criticised for assuming that cultures are both unchanging and homogenous. However, cultures are complex, variable and contested. As Donnelly (2003) states, cultures are fluid complexes of inter-subjective meaning and practices. In Case 3.2 about the older man who had been vegan wanting to eat meat, the contested meanings are evident in how to interpret what may be a counter-culture of adopting a vegan diet and how differing interpretations of client autonomy may interface with how the well-being of the client is negotiated.

In immersing ourselves in human rights, the question of self-determination is one that is to the forefront. Bowles et al. (2006) speak of the individual's right to self-determination being based on the consideration of individuals as free beings who are able to take their own decisions. As demonstrated in Cases 3.1 (about the man in the psychiatric hospital) and 3.2 (about the reluctant vegan) this right cannot be taken for granted and, as happened in 3.2, may require external formal intervention. In Case 3.1 what becomes evident is the limit to self-determination in a securitised site of social control and how this creates tension for the human rights social worker. Can the right to self-determination ever be waived? In the ideal practice setting, the answer should be a resounding 'no'. As early as the 1960s, Biestek (1961) referred to self-determination as one of the most important principles of professional practice, something that may be seen as in violation in these two cases.

Another question that may confront social workers is the issue of rights and responsibilities – but with vulnerable people we see that the 'responsibility' issue may be privileged particularly for people forced onto social security provision. As funding cuts take hold in many countries, ostensibly as a result of the 'global economic crisis', it is likely that this issue will revive in intensity. The other human rights perspective that comes to the forefront is respect – a concept integral to the question of rights as the title to this chapter suggests. To some degree, a human rights approach also dispels the notion of 'tolerance', for if human rights are for all, then respect for people as fellow human beings goes beyond tolerating difference to affirming difference. Clark with Asquith (1985: 29) place respect for human rights to the forefront in their list of typical clients' rights drawn from the literature, of which the following is a selection:

- To be treated as an end.
- To be accepted for what one is.
- To be treated as a unique individual.
- To be treated within principles of honesty, openness and non-deception.
- To have information given to the worker in the course of social work treatment treated as confidential.

Some of the examples outlined in this chapter highlight the uniqueness of the individual and the desire to be accepted for what one is, particularly Cases 3.1 and 3.2. The right to honesty and non-deception, however, are somewhat vexed in the other two case studies and need to be read alongside the contest between universal principles and cultural relativism. If we use these rights to consider Case 3.4 in particular, which focuses on research in India, we need to go beyond the espoused principles. This case also raises uncomfortable questions that arise in cultural settings other than our own and where we may approach social work practice with our own ethical lens that may not apply in the same way in other contexts. We share Ife's (2008) position in stating that the key to dealing with cultural difference is the capacity to look critically at all cultural traditions and to see human rights as important in all countries, while seeing how they are contextualised differently. More controversially, Rachels (2003) states that relativism prevents us from imposing our own values on other cultural groups (as in Case 3.3, set in Vietnam) but could also lead to inaction in the face of what may constitute human rights violations (see Case 3.4, set in India).

Applying human rights

Each of the contributors has extended their practice lens to contemplate how a social work approach reveals understandings that can be applied. In each case the complexities and contradictions of social work are to the forefront and in most cases more questions are raised than answers provided.

As the cases so aptly demonstrate, human rights for social workers are not a mere grand plan or unachievable aspiration. Ensuring the application of a combined human rights and ethical framework to every method and field of practice can encourage the profession to pave the way through complexities and contradictions.

Human rights and social work ethics are intertwined, as well as linking with concepts of social justice. A human rights framework forms a solid moral base for the profession, reflecting a concern that all persons should enjoy basic rights (Dewees 2005).

References

Biestek, F. (1961) *The Casework Relationship*, London: Allen and Unwin.

Black, B. (2008) 'Empowering and rights-based approaches to working with older people', in J. Allan, L. Briskman and B. Pease (eds) *Critical Social Work: Theories and Practices for a Socially Just World*, Sydney: Allen and Unwin.

Bowles, W., Collingridge, M., Curry, S. and Valentine, B. (2006) *Ethical Practice in Social Work: An Applied Approach*, Maidenhead, UK: Open University Press/McGraw-Hill.

Briskman, L. (2007a) 'Menschenrechte und soziale Arbeit – eine globale Perspektive' [Human rights and social work – a global perspective] in L. Wagner and R. Lutz, (eds) *Internationale Perspektiven Sozialer Arbeit*, Frankfurt am Main: Verlag für Interkulturelle Kommunikation.

Briskman, L. (2007b), *Social Work with Indigenous Communities*, Sydney: The Federation Press.

Cemlyn, S. (2008) 'Human rights and gypsies and travellers: an exploration of the application of a human rights perspective to social work with a minority community in Britain', *British Journal of Social Work*, 38(1): 153–173.

Clark, C. with Asquith, S. (1985) *Social Work and Social Philosophy*, London: Routledge and Kegan Paul.

Dewees, M. (2005) *Contemporary Social Work Practice*, Boston: McGraw-Hill.

Dominelli, L. (1998) 'Social work research: contested knowledge for practice', in R. Adams, L. Dominelli and M. Payne (eds) *Social Work Futures: Crossing Boundaries, Transforming Practice*, Basingstoke, UK: Palgrave Macmillan.

Donnelly, J. (2003) *Universal Human Rights in Theory and Practice*, 2nd edition, New York: Cornell University Press.

Fiske, L. and Briskman, L. (2008) 'Teaching human rights at university: critical pedagogy in action', in B. Offord and C. Newell (eds) *Activating Human Rights in Education: Exploration, Innovation and Transformation*, Canberra: Australian College of Educators.

Ife, J. (2001) *Human Rights and Social Work: Towards Rights-Based Practice*, Cambridge: Cambridge University Press.

Ife, J. (2008) *Human Rights and Social Work: Towards Rights-Based Practice*, revised edition, Cambridge: Cambridge University Press.

International Federation of Social Workers and International Association of Schools of Social Work (2004) *Ethics in Social Work: Statement of Principles*, Berne: IFSW and IASSW.

Nipperess, S. and Briskman L. (2009) 'Promoting a human rights perspective on critical social work', in J. Allan, L. Briskman and B. Pease (eds) *Critical Social Work: Theories and Practices for a Socially Just World*, Sydney: Allen and Unwin.

Rachels, J. (2003) *The Elements of Moral Philosophy*, 4th edition, New York: McGraw-Hill.

Reichert, E. (2003) *Social Work and Human Rights: A Foundation for Policy and Practice*, New York: Columbia University Press.

Rioux, M. and Zubrow, E. (2001) 'Social disability in the public good,' in D. Drache (ed.) *The Market or the Public Domain: Global Governance and the Asymmetry of Power*, London: Routledge.

United Nations (1948) *Universal Declaration of Human Rights*, www.un.org/en/documents/udhr/index.shtml, accessed October 2010.

Case 3.1   Issues of choice and coercion: working in a psychiatric hospital in the USA

Introduction

This case, written by a female social worker, took place in Virginia, in the south eastern United States. At the time, in order to be involuntarily hospitalised a client would need to be: 1) a danger to him- or herself; 2) a danger to others; or 3) substantively unable to take care of her- or himself as a result of the mental illness. If one or more of these criteria were met, the client could be detained (under a temporary detention order or TDO) at a psychiatric hospital for a short period of time (usually not more than 72 hours) for observation. At the end of this time a commitment hearing would be conducted. If a committed client refused medication, then medication could be court-ordered, a procedure called an order to treat. Medications mentioned here include mood stabilising medication (such as Depakote and Lithium, typically used to treat bipolar disorder) and anti-psychotic medication (such as Haldol) used to control symptoms of psychosis.

The case

When I was working as an in-patient psychiatric social worker on a 30-bed hospital unit located in a rural area I encountered a client similar to the one described here, whom I have called Carson. At this time, I had been out of my Master of Social Work programme for about three years and often found myself questioning the line between persuasion and coercion in encouraging clients to take their psychotropic/psychiatric medications.

The morning after Carson's admission, the nurses were upset with his behaviour of the night before. He had written in faeces on the wall, stripped and been sexually and physically aggressive when the nurses tried to give him medication. The nurses forcibly injected Carson with Haldol after he slapped the medications out of a nurse's hand, on the grounds that this met the criterion of 'danger to others'. The hope in administering the anti-psychotic medication (Haldol) was to decrease his aggressive behaviour and help stabilise his functioning.

Carson was a 40-year-old man with a history of bipolar disorder. Three years before admission to this hospital, he had been hospitalised in a state psychiatric facility. Carson was a bright and highly educated man who worked for a prestigious company in a nearby city. This hospitalisation resulted from a *Temporary Detention Order (TDO)* prompted by his 'bizarre behaviour' in the community and at his workplace – including dancing in the street and other manic symptoms. Throughout his hospital stay, Carson maintained that he was not bizarre but rather 'high-spirited' and creative. He felt that others were unable to tolerate any kind of deviant behaviour.

The hearing resulted in Carson's involuntary commitment to the hospital. The commitment order requires the client to remain hospitalised until discharged by a psychiatrist. During the hearing, Carson agreed with his diagnosis of bipolar disorder. He felt he did have a 'chemical imbalance' and for this reason had already agreed to take Lithium because it 'was a natural salt his body lacked'. He refused any type of anti-psychotic drug because of the side effects he had experienced when taking them briefly in the past. He also felt he was oriented to reality and did not need other medications.

A dilemma in working with Carson was the result of the psychiatrist's opinion that Carson would benefit from a low dose of a neuroleptic, in addition to adding Depakote (a mood stabiliser like Lithium) to the prescribed Lithium. Carson would not hear of it. The psychiatrist charged me with convincing Carson to take these additional medications. The psychiatrist made it clear that Carson's continued refusal of the medications would result in an Order to Treat. The Order to Treat was a dilemma for me as a social worker in this hospital setting. It seemed to me that a client should have the last say about whether he or she takes a medication. If the client refuses the prescribed medication, then a member of the nursing staff gives the medication by injection while the client is restrained.

Carson had never stopped taking the Lithium. It was obvious that Lithium alone was not alleviating his current symptoms. My dilemma was whether it was my responsibility to inform him of the potential benefits of the additional medications and let him make an informed decision. However, I questioned whether he could make an informed decision considering his unstable mood state.

Complicating the dilemma for me was Carson's threat of legal action. He was enraged that he had been forcibly injected with Haldol earlier in his hospital stay. He solicited the involvement of other patients on the unit in his outrage against staff members. The unit took on a very uncomfortable 'us and them' atmosphere between staff and patients. Meanwhile, the psychiatrist believed that I was being 'sucked in' by Carson since I expressed reluctance to carry out her recommendations for medication compliance. I became tired of Carson accusing me of being a 'lackey for the system' and found myself wishing he would simply be quiet. This flew in the face of my professional values of self-determination. I had always been passionate about client self-determination. I noticed that the other staff had little of my own conflict about this situation with Carson and clearly saw him as 'crazy' and in desperate need of medication.

After a week or so, the psychiatrist agreed that Carson, now improved on the combination of Depakote and Lithium, which he had agreed to take, could probably convince the judge presiding over the Order to Treat that he did not pose a threat without the anti-psychotic medication. She stated that 'next time' we would need to get the Order early on and avoid the dialogue and argument with him. The doctor then discharged Carson. For several weeks following his discharge Carson called and sent hostile letters every few days about his treatment by the hospital staff. In his communications, he singled me out as one of the worst offenders and sent me insulting notes. This was a blow to me, as I believed that I had advocated on his behalf with the psychiatrist for his right to refuse the additional medications. I had spent a great amount of time with him. I felt muddled and irritated, and questioned what other or different actions I could have taken in the situation.

My experience working with Carson has been one of those cases I have often referred back to both in reflection and as part of my teaching. My reactions to working with him have illustrated for me that some of our most uncomfortable practice experiences can actually be our most fertile learning opportunities. I was extremely saddened several years later to learn of Carson's death. He died after a physical encounter with police that occurred during a screening, once again, for involuntary hospitalisation.

Commentary 1

DONNA HARRINGTON

The social worker working with Carson in a psychiatric hospital in Virginia faced an ethical dilemma with a number of contextual factors that complicated the decision-making process. As described in the case, the major dilemma revolves around Carson's right to self-determination (i.e., refusing to take the prescribed medication) and the psychiatrist's charge to the social worker to 'convince Carson to take the additional medications'.

Clients' rights to self-determination

In the United States, and many Western countries, self-determination is a highly valued right. The International Federation of Social Workers (IFSW) and International Association of Schools of Social Work (IASSW) emphasise clients' right to self-determination, stating that 'social workers should respect and promote people's right to make their own choices and decisions, irrespective of their values and life choices, provided this does not threaten the rights and legitimate interests of others' (IFSW and IASSW 2004: Principle 4.1.1). In the United States, the Code of Ethics of the National Association of Social Workers (NASW 2008: Standard 1.02) also emphasises self-determination, stating that:

> Social workers respect and promote the right of clients to self-deter-
> mination and assist clients in their efforts to identify and clarify their
> goals. Social workers may limit clients' right to self-determination
> when, in the social worker's professional judgment, clients' actions
> or potential actions pose a serious, foreseeable, and imminent risk to
> themselves or others.

Both codes of ethics emphasise self-determination, but with limits if others' rights are threatened or there is an imminent risk of harm for the client or others. This suggests that protection of life may be a higher priority than protection of self-determination.

As the social worker in this case noted, Carson should have the right to decide which, if any, medications he would take. However, this right may be limited if he is not capable of making this decision or his choice not to take the medication will threaten others' rights or safety. The social worker in this case states that 'my dilemma was whether it was my responsibility to inform him of the potential benefits of the additional medications and let him make an informed decision. However, I questioned whether he could make an informed decision considering his unstable mood state.' I'm not sure there is an ethical dilemma here. If Carson is capable of making an informed decision then the social worker should inform him of the benefits *and risks* of the additional medications so that he can make an informed decision. However, if he is not capable of making an informed decision, then someone else should have the legal responsibility to do so. The case does not state whether Carson is competent to make decisions. Further, 'Carson's involuntary commitment to the hospital' suggests that there was a threat of harm to himself or others. The right to self-determination may be limited when decision-making ability is impaired or there is a threat of harm to self or others.

The social worker in this case does not appear to be questioning whether Carson should have been involuntarily committed; and it appears that there was some risk to others, suggesting that Carson's right to self-determination may be limited. But, limiting a client's right to self-determination, even if required to protect life, should not be taken lightly and the right should be restored as soon as the client is able to participate in the decision-making process and no longer poses a threat to self or others.

Contextual factors

This case was complicated by several contextual factors because the social worker was caught between the client's wishes and someone else's charge, which raises the question of to whom the social worker owes loyalty – the client, her employer, or herself? The loyalty owed to the client is clear in that social workers are obligated to promote clients' well-being. Loyalty to an employer or colleagues (i.e., the hospital and psychiatrist) is usually of a lower priority than that owed to the client, but is still an important consideration. And, finally, the social worker owes loyalty to herself in terms of maintaining professional values and ethics, as well as personal safety. While some may suggest that clients' well-being should come first no matter what, it may not be reasonable to expect that a social worker will always be able or willing to promote clients' well-being at the risk of her own job or personal safety. As the author notes, the situation was also complicated by 'Carson's threat of legal action', which may have presented both financial and professional risks for the social worker. Although these issues are not strictly part of the ethical dilemma, they do provide the context in which decisions have to be made, and as such need to be acknowledged. It is much easier to consider this ethical dilemma when one is not personally placed between a client and a supervisor or colleague while being threatened with legal action.

Conclusion

When the client's right to self-determination has been limited, the question for the social worker becomes what he or she can do to best promote the client's well-being in that situation. As the social worker did in this case, it is important to advocate for the client's rights and to continue to involve the client in the decision-making process to the greatest extent possible. Finally, it is important to work with the client and others to restore the client's right to self-determination as soon as possible.

References

International Federation of Social Workers and International Association of Schools of Social Work (2004) *Ethics in Social Work, Statement of Principles*, Berne: IFSW and IASSW (available at: www.ifsw.org).

National Association of Social Workers (2008) *Code of Ethics*, Washington, DC: NASW (available at: www.naswdc.org/pubs/code/code.asp).

Donna Harrington is Professor and Ph.D. Program Director, University of Maryland School of Social Work, Baltimore, MD, USA; she has a Ph.D. in Applied Developmental Psychology.

Commentary 2

SIU-MAN NG

A number of dilemmas involving core professional values became highly intensified in the course of working with Carson, who was seemingly in a manic episode and was involuntarily admitted to a psychiatric hospital. Carson was in an unstable mental state such that his decision-making ability and self-inhibition function were significantly impaired.

Respect for self-determination and the exceptions

A critical factor here was whether the client, Carson, could make an informed decision on taking medications in his first week of admission to hospital. If Carson's mental state was so unstable that his decision-making ability was severely impaired, it did not make any sense and was unethical to 'convince' him to take neuroleptic medication. Therefore the psychiatrist's request for the social worker's help in 'convincing' Carson was logically at fault in the first place. The psychiatrist's statement that Carson's continued refusal of the medications would result in an *Order to Treat* was essentially a threat, which could be regarded as professional ethical misconduct. It could also be interpreted as a tactic to avoid going through the proper legal procedures of obtaining an *Order to Treat*. If the psychiatrist firmly believed that the neuroleptic was absolutely necessary, she should have taken the case to a formal hearing in which Carson would be adequately represented and independent opinions would be considered.

A central spirit of mental health law is the protection of the rights of psychiatric patients, at the same time as some of their rights to self-determination are being limited in exceptional situations. An important role of the social worker is to ensure that the spirit of mental health law is understood, appreciated and respected. Tactics of bypassing legal procedures should be scrutinised, questioned and challenged. While some colleagues in the mental health team may consider those tactics as 'shortcuts' or 'clever ways for minimising administrative tasks', they should be educated on the deeper impacts of those acts, in particular in depriving clients of the protection of their human rights under the law.

Accountability to the client versus accountability to the multidisciplinary team

It is a core social work value that accountability to the client is the first priority. In the context of a medical setting, a social worker is a member of the multidisciplinary team and has accountability to it. Meanwhile, the social worker to some extent also represents an outside agent with an emphasis on humanity and social justice. These different roles and account-abilities are often in conflict. In reading the case report, I strongly felt the social worker's resistance to the psychiatrist's request. At the same time, I could also feel the social worker's lack of support and sense of helplessness because she seemed to be the only one in the team who suffered from intense internal struggles. To her further dismay, it was her who was singled out by Carson in the subsequent hostile phone calls and letters he made after discharge. I could imagine that it had been an extremely difficult time for the social worker. If I were the social worker, I might have suffered confusion over core social work values and ethical principles. While I was reading the case report, I was deeply impressed by the social worker's reflection on her practice and persistence in holding onto her core beliefs.

In face of ethical dilemmas, a social worker is inevitably forced to take sides among conflicting roles and accountabilities. This can be extremely tough, and thus highlights the importance of continued clinical supervision from an independent source. This point is also relevant from an ethical perspective, because agencies do have a duty to ensure their staff work and behave professionally and ethically. Regular access to clinical supervision is especially essential for clinical social workers because of their close working relationships with the clients. In-depth reflection with proper facilitation in a safe environment is highly desirable.

Siu-man Ng, Ph.D., is Assistant Professor in the Department of Social Work and Social Administration, The University of Hong Kong. He is Chinese, and grew up and was educated in Hong Kong. He has a professional background in psychiatric social work and Chinese medicine. With a close historical tie with the UK, the Mental Health Ordinance of Hong Kong resembles the Mental Health Act of the UK.

Questions for discussion about Case 3.1

1 The main ethical focus of this case is a psychiatric patient's rights to self-determination. What do you think is meant by 'self-determination' and why is it regarded as so important in Western societies?

2 What other ethical issues does this case raise? What might be the perspectives of other participants in the scenario, apart from the social worker and Carson?

3 If you had been the social worker's supervisor, how might you have supported her in handling this difficult case?

Case study 3.2

Case 3.2 The reluctant vegan: the case of an older man in a Swedish care home

Introduction

This case comes from Sweden and is about a man with Alzheimer's disease who was living in a residential care home. In Sweden, care homes tend to be small units. Care homes are all publicly financed and may be run by municipalities, non-profit and for-profit organisations. Residential homes for older people are usually managed by social workers or nurses or other staff with different qualifications, and staffed by social care workers. Each resident has a key worker who coordinates their care. As far as possible the care workers try to respect the choices of the residents, insofar as they are able to express their preferences.

The case: whether to allow an inveterate vegan to eat meat?[1]

A 75-year-old man, who had been deeply involved in the vegan movement for many years, fell ill with Alzheimer's disease and was placed in a

---

1 This case has been adapted from the Akademikerförbundet SSR website. We are grateful to Akademikerförbundet SSR for giving permission to use it.

residential home, where in accordance with his previous habits he was served vegan meals. One day, by mistake, he happened to eat a portion of meatballs, potatoes, brown sauce and lingon berries that was intended for another resident. He enjoyed it very much and at the next meal noticed for the first time that he was being served different food to all the others. The care workers persuaded him to eat his vegan meal, but the next day he refused point-blank to eat 'any special muck that's only for me'.

His key worker discussed the situation with his wife, who in no uncertain terms expressly forbade the staff to give him anything but vegan food. She insisted that it was against his (and her) convictions to eat meat or 'warmed-over dead body parts', as she put it. The staff tried to comply, but encountered vociferous protest at each meal from the man, who sometimes, with triumph and great delight, managed to appropriate food left over by someone else at the table.

The head of the unit and the staff were not sure how to handle this. Should they allow him to eat meat? What should they tell his wife?

Afterword

This case is real and was analysed by the Ethical Committee of the Swedish National Board of Health and Welfare. The committee came to the conclusion that the staff should respect the man's wish to choose his own food. The fact that previously he had a certain opinion (for vegan food) did not prevent him from changing his mind later in life.

Commentary 1

TITTI FRÄNKEL AND ERIK BLENNBERGER

The right to decide about your own life and to change your mind

The case of the vegan man at an old-people's home who gets a taste of meat brings forward principles of self-determination and individual freedom – which relate to the right of each human being to make decisions and take actions that concern their own lives. Corresponding to these rights there are obligations on others. In a home for older people, the residents should have the space and the resources for self-determination, and should be able to 'be themselves'. From the account of this case, it is clear that the man's previous decision to be a vegan was honoured at the residential home with regard to his diet. He was only served vegan food. Then, by chance, he gained a taste for other types of food and wished to change his diet. He wanted to have meat. Are there any reasons to deny him this?

Conceivable reasons to prevent the man from eating meat

Could the strong objection of the man's wife be such a reason? If the man turns into a meat-eater she might change her attitude towards him completely. There is a risk that he begins to appear revolting to her and becomes a person she no longer wishes to meet. Is it worth risking the relationship with the wife only because the man would like to have meat? The man may not understand this risk, since his judgement and capability to make decisions are strongly reduced by his illness. However, should the staff at the residential home merely establish how the man's wife judges the situation and act on her request? Should there not be attempts to increase the understanding of the choice that the man has made, and of his mental situation? Furthermore, regardless of this, why should she decide about his eating habits?

Are there any other reasons to deny the man food that contains meat? How would we look upon his wish to have meat if he occasionally had what are called 'moments of clarity', which are common at least in the initial stages of dementia? If, in a moment of clarity with regard to his disease, he were to understand that he actually had changed his diet, it might generate a deep remorse, maybe self-contempt. Is it worth putting him at that risk? Moreover, what if, in an instant of soundness like this, he clarifies that he never ever wants to eat meat any more? Is it then possible to refer to this statement if he later, in a more confused state, changes his mind again?

These arguments, which involve the reactions of the wife and the – probably painful – experience of the man as a meat eater, are all about judging consequences. At a home for older people, arguments like this do sometimes have to be weighed against each other. They concern conditions that improve the quality of life of the residents. However, in such considerations, there is also a danger of (an overriding) paternalism on the part of staff and relatives, where the requests of the elderly are not honoured.

Two lines of arguments for principles of freedom and self-determination

When this case was discussed at the Ethical Committee of the Swedish Board on Health and Welfare many of the points discussed above were made. However, the overwhelming majority considered that the man's right to self-determination had to be respected. Therefore, if he requested to eat meat, he should be allowed to do so. The right to freedom and self-determination are strong ethical principles that also have robust support in Swedish legislation, not least in the field of care of the elderly.

If we take the principle of self-determination, two lines of argument may be taken to support this. One option, from a deontological perspective, is to perceive self-determination as intrinsically valuable and as constituting a fundamental human right. Nonetheless, there may be certain limitations. A person must not use his or her freedom to prevent the freedom of others. Another potential limitation is when there is a risk of the person harming him- or herself (a person may be mentally ill or in a state of shock and lack the capability to make decisions). However, none of these reservations is valid in this case. The decision to eat meat does not constrain the freedom of anyone else; and the man is not in danger of harming himself by eating meat.

Another line of argument for self-determination is utilitarian. The main message here is that the best consequences are usually gained when people are left to decide in matters that pertain to their own lives. The best decisions are made in this way. Even if we sometimes make incorrect decisions we would feel deeply uncomfortable if others were to govern the decisions of our lives. We would also become diminished as human beings if we were deprived the rights of independence in relation to important issues. The right of self-determination is seen as an instrumental value and is important because it yields the best consequences.

How we interpret the principle of self-determination – as a value in its own right or as an instrumental value – will give different conditions for the discussion, although the conclusions on how finally to act may be identical.

The right to eat meatballs – from different points of departure

Regardless of how we argue with regard to the principle of self-determination, the conclusion in this specific case is the same – the man should have a right to his meatballs. If the principle of self-determination is given an intrinsic value and is seen from a deontological point of view, there is not much room for uncertainty. However, if the principle of self-determination is observed from a utilitarian outlook, the consideration often will be more ambiguous. Other aspects have to be taken into account, not least the attitude of the wife and how this attitude affects the man. Using a judgement based on consequentialism, it seems to be slightly easier to consider the different nuances of a problem and to retain a particular degree of uncertainty. It becomes somewhat less difficult to recognise that there are some reasons that speak against the decisions that people have made – although these reasons are not strong enough to change the view in this case that the man should have a right to choose meatballs for dinner.

Titti Fränkel is Development Manager at Akademikerförbundet SSR, which is a professional organisation and a union for social workers in Sweden.
Erik Blennberger is Associate Professor, Doctor of Divinity and Director of Research at the Institute for Organisational and Worklife Ethics, Ersta Sköndal University College, Sweden. He is also a member of the Swedish Ethical Board on Health and Welfare, author of several books on ethics, and author of several ethical codes for different professions and organisations.

Commentary 2

HILDE LINDEMANN

In 'Freedom of the will and the concept of a person', the philosopher Harry Frankfurt (1988) argues that the difference between a morally responsible person and a 'wanton' (his examples are young children and severely cognitively impaired adults) is that persons do not just have desires – they have desires about their desires. That is, they can evaluate the things they want, decide whether they *want* to want them, and act accordingly. 'Wantons,' by contrast, are not capable of making these evaluative judgements, so they simply act on whatever desires they happen to have.

As the man in this case suffers from a dementia that has progressed to the point where he can no longer be cared for at home, it seems highly probable that, in Frankfurt's terms, he is a wanton, no longer able to control his desire to eat meat by wanting not to have that desire. Because he is not free to choose which desires to act on, it makes no more sense to hold him responsible for his actions than it does a drug addict, a toddler, or a chipmunk. Instead, we take a different attitude toward him, managing or handling or humouring him, without holding him to the same standards of morality to which we hold ordinary adults.

It does not take Harry Frankfurt, though, to tell us that a man with well-advanced Alzheimer's disease is no longer morally responsible. The more interesting part of Frankfurt's analysis is that it helps us see why we should not agree with the Ethical Committee's view that the man has just changed his mind about eating meat. Changing one's mind, especially about something that involves a moral commitment, is not simply a matter of now choosing X when you previously chose Y. You also have to repudiate your commitment to Y (Nelson 2009). When a person is demented enough to lose his ability to want what he wants, however, he is no longer in a position to repudiate his commitments – to say to himself that on reflection he finds them less worthy than he previously did.

If this is right, then our reluctant vegan probably is not capable of changing his mind. His previously formed evaluative judgement still deserves respect, though, because in making it and then sticking to it for so much of his life, the man defined himself morally: the story of his commitment to veganism played some kind of role in his identity. We might not know exactly how much of a role, of course, because we do not know how centrally the commitment to veganism figured in who he was. But his wife knows, and it may be her sense of his identity that now motivates her to insist that he not be given any meat. She might be making up for his inability to want what he wants by regulating his desires for him in accordance with her understanding of who he is.

But then the question arises of whether he still is that person. One of the most devastating features of a progressive dementia is that it gradually disintegrates the person, leaving loved ones struggling to keep up with the changes. That is all the more reason for those who have a long, shared history with the person to resist the damage as long as possible rather than cooperate with the disease's inexorable obliteration of the self. The wife, therefore, may be trying to make sure that, as long as possible, her husband's actions be guided to conform with the identity to which he has, by his choices, contributed over all the years of his life.

I want to resist the idea that people are successions of person-slices, with old selves dropping away as new ones form. It is certainly true that some of the stories that constitute a person's identity no longer have the same salience they once did, and new stories must be added to reflect the way the person changes over time. But the whole messy tissue of identity-constituting stories attaches to the person like a continually growing comet's tail, and cannot just be sheared off as the person's self diminishes into dementia. Who the person has been is a part of who they are now – maybe even the most important part.

Still, we must not let the comet's tail wag the comet – or at least, not altogether. So much has changed for this man that it may not seem reasonable to hold him to moral commitments that he no longer understands. There is so little left to him that it might seem cruel to deprive him of the few pleasures that yet remain, and I doubt any of us would fault the wife for permitting him to indulge in his carnivorous desires. Indeed, the fault-finding is much more apt to lie on the other side of the question, which is why I have taken such pains to try to show why her insistence on keeping him from indulging could be reasonable too.

On a practical level, it might help if the husband could be fed in his room, where he would not know what the others are eating, at least until he is too demented to care. If the staff cannot manage that, though, and the man is made seriously unhappy by being denied meat, the wife may have to consider how important it is for him to remain true to the principles he has lived by. It may be very important indeed, but perhaps it might not matter as much as his present distress. It is not a decision she can make by herself, as the staff members are involved as well, but because her life has presumably been inextricably intertwined with his for a very long time, she has more at stake here than they do. She, after all, is the only one in a position to consider what he would have done, had their roles been reversed and he been the one to decide what she should eat. And that way of thinking about it might, at the end of the day, be everybody's best option.

References

Frankfurt, H. G. (1988) 'Freedom of the will and the concept of a person', in H. G. Frankfurt (ed.), *The Importance of What We Care About*, New York: Cambridge University Press.

Nelson, J. L. (2009) 'Alzheimer's disease and socially extended mentation', *Metaphilosophy* 40(3/4): 462–474.

Hilde Lindemann is Professor of Philosophy, Michigan State University, USA.

Questions for discussion about Case 3.2

1 What are the main differences in the approach to this case offered in the two commentaries?

2 Who do you think has the *right* to decide whether or not the man eats meat? Who has the *responsibility* to decide?

3   How much do you think it matters whether or not the man eats meatballs – to the man himself, to his wife and to the staff of the home?

Case 3.3   Social work in Vietnam: a Dutch student's perspective

Introduction

This case is written by a Dutch social work student, while undertaking fieldwork practice in a hospital in a town in the centre of Vietnam. This town is located near the former border between North and South Vietnam. During the Vietnam War, this was the part that suffered the most from bombings and chemicals such as 'agent orange', and it is still considered as a poor area of Vietnam.

Study programmes in social work have only recently been developed in Vietnam, with officially recognised Bachelor's degrees starting in 2004. There is a small group of graduate social workers active in Vietnam, who sometimes work for NGOs, but mostly they work independently because of the few available social work jobs. The practical experience gained during the study is limited so when the students graduate their main contribution to organisations is theoretical knowledge. From the point of view of the organisations, theoretical knowledge of social work is perhaps not attractive enough to hire a social worker.

The case

I am based at a rehabilitation department of a hospital in Vietnam, studying for my minor subject: 'International social work and community development'. I am in my final year as a social work student in the Netherlands and chose this placement because of my international interest. I am in Vietnam to research the role social work can play in the context of physical rehabilitation. In the hospital where the rehabilitation department is situated, one social worker is present in the team of rehabilitation caregivers. This social worker gained knowledge about social work through the internet.

Every week the staff (physiotherapists) from the rehabilitation department where I work visit one or more patients in the field. The goals of these visits are to gain information about the current daily life activities of the patients, to answer questions the patients have and to examine their current physical health. The reason I am involved in these visits is to give the staff some advice and help on how to use social work aspects during the conversations.

This case is about Trung, an eight-year-old boy who suffers from Duchenne Muscular Dystrophy (DMD, a severe form of muscular dystrophy characterised by rapid progression of muscle degeneration). In advance, I was told that Trung is not able to walk or stand and that besides DMD he has problems with his lungs, which makes breathing hard sometimes.

When we entered the house the first thing I noticed was the boy: to me he looked really weak and skinny. He sat in a wheelchair that was obviously too big for him – his arms couldn't reach the wheels. The boy was writing in a notebook on a little tableau made on the wheelchair.

As we sat down, the parents started talking. The mother informed us, full of pride, that Trung had won the first prize in his writing class; his handwriting was the most beautiful out of a class of 30 children. The mother told us that every day she took her son to school on the motorbike, with her husband coming with them and leaving them at school for the morning. She has to stay there every day because during the classes she needs to help her son with his physical problems. The teacher does not have enough time for that and is not educated in caring for disabled children. In the afternoon Trung and his mother come home, then Trung can start on his homework.

One of the physiotherapists gave Trung a compliment on his writing and drawing: 'It looks really beautiful', he said. The boy smiled for one second and then looked with concentration again at his notebook. I asked the boy what his favourite subject at school was, he answered, 'Mathematics.' In response to a question about what he wanted to be when he grew up, he did not have an answer. He thought about it for a long time, then sighed and said: 'I don't know yet.'

I asked Trung if he liked to play with other children, and he answered very enthusiastically: 'Yes.' He said his favourite activities were drawing and playing games, and that he often watched the other children playing soccer. I asked him if it was difficult for him to watch them play, and he replied that it made him sad.

Trung's parents own a farm where they grow rice, potatoes and tea. The products are mainly for their own use, but when there is enough left the mother goes to the market to sell the rest. Financially it is not easy for the family; because of the care Trung needs the mother is not able to have a job outside of the house. Trung is their only child and besides Trung's grandmother, who lives with them, there is no support for the family.

One of the physiotherapists asked if they had any questions for us. The mother wanted to know when there would be an improvement in Trung's physical condition. The physiotherapist said he did not know, but that Trung had to keep doing his exercises. As a final question I asked Trung if he had any worries. He said he had a lot of pain and that he was worried about his health. We thanked the family for having us as visitors and then we left to go back to the rehabilitation department.

Back at the rehabilitation department I wanted to do an evaluation of the visit. We talked about Trung's situation and I asked the staff if any improvement is possible when someone suffers from Duchenne Muscular Dystrophy. They said improvement is not possible and that because of the lung problems Trung has, it is a possibility that he will not have a long life ahead of him. I asked them if the parents and Trung knew this. The rehabilitation staff replied that it was better for them not to know, because if they did, then they would feel sad until the time came for Trung.

My opinion

This approach is in contradiction with my social work ethics. But the staff explained to me that this is their way of working and it is better for the boy not to feel sad, because in their opinion that might increase the weakness of the muscles. Another argument for them not to tell the truth about the prognosis was the quality of the boy's life. According to the medical staff, if Trung knew that he would die, for example, in less than a year, he would spend the rest of his life miserable knowing that.

From my point of view as a social worker, this could not be determined by the medical staff for as far as we know the boy could spend his last months perfectly happy. And even if he was not happy, is it bad to feel sad? Is not feeling sad a part of life as well? Do professionals have the right or power to prevent someone from being sad? By not telling him and his family the truth, the possibility to have a normal grieving process and to be able to overcome the pain which comes along with the prognosis is taken from the boy and his family. It got me wondering whether this is a difference in intercultural sensitivity or a lack of knowledge about coping with psychological problems.

The medical staff were very curious about the Western way of handling this type of situation. I explained to them that in the Netherlands we try to be very open and honest about a patient's medical situation. The medical staff were very interested in learning more about this – how to tell 'bad news', and how to overcome or accept bad news.

After talking to many Vietnamese people about this, it seemed that the approach of the medical staff was based on a combination of lack of knowledge, not knowing how to bring 'bad news', and was also culturally linked. They told me that it was perfectly normal for them not to be honest when giving diagnoses or prognoses. Often family members do know the truth, but patients themselves do not. This shocked me, because in my belief, which is similar to the average Western belief, every person deserves to know the truth about their medical situation.

Commentary 1

NGUYEN THI THAI LAN

Background: social work in Vietnam

Since 2004, social work has been introduced as an official training field in Vietnam at the college (three years of training) and university levels (four years of training). Only after 2004 was an official Bachelor's degree in social work offered. However, the first university that provided social work training was Hochiminh Open University in the early 1990s, located in Hochiminh City (the south of Vietnam). This university training programme was called 'Women's Studies'. In the north, the University of Labour and Social Affairs (originally called the College of Labour and Social Affairs) was the first training institution that provided a three-year social work training programme in the 'Sociology' field. All of these programmes provide a certain amount of time for practice, although practice was given a very limited amount of time at the beginning. Due to the fact that social work was not recognised officially as an occupation until 2010, social work graduates have great difficulty in finding jobs. However, they can apply to work for NGOs or international NGOs, government agencies in charge of labour, invalids and social affairs from commune to central level (Department of Labour, Invalids and Social Affairs, Social Protection Centres), and other small private open houses. The above information shows that social work in Vietnam is a very new field and it is just in the very early stage of development. Therefore, it is very difficult to acquire a perfect professional environment for practice.

The story behind the different contexts

It is understandable that the author of the case had the feeling of shock when she was in the situation in Vietnam. In order to explain the situation, it is better to look at the contexts – the two different contexts the author has experienced. First is the context of the developed country (the Netherlands) where she was born, grew up and had her professional social work training. As a professionally trained Western social work student, the situation in Vietnam would be very strange. It might seem unacceptable if the professionals are not honest in telling their patients and clients about the details of their severe medical and social circumstances. However, in the other context (Vietnam), where the author had her short practice, the picture is so different. In Vietnam, at the time of the author's practice placement, the concept of social work is still very new and it is understood mostly as charity work. As can be seen in the case, even though there is a staff member calling her-/himself a 'social worker', there was no such title in the official job list until 2010. Besides that, apparently the knowledge and skills s/he learnt had been gained only from the internet. Thus, it can be said that in the second context (Vietnam), professional social work has not been fully introduced and implemented. This explains why decisions and actions occur that would be regarded as inappropriate in relation to the ethical principles of professional social work.

Nevertheless, even if the medical staff did tell all the family members in this case about the real and sad situation of the eight-year-old child, in this context (Vietnam) it is predicted that the situation would be worse for the family. Experience with many other cases in Vietnam suggests that either the child would not cooperate in treatment or the parents would be so sad that the miserable family environment would affect the treatment efforts and the level of support from family members. They would lose their hope. This approach is because of lack of knowledge, as the author of the case has identified. However, the question still remains: 'Is it an ethical decision to do something that you can see is harmful to your patients or that will create another problem?' The answer would be that, if you do not know how to help your patients to cope, it is better not to make any decision. So our task as social workers is to provide and share adequate knowledge and skills to help those professionals to choose the right ethical decision. It is important to start with the context where people themselves come from.

Culture and professional ethics

The second issue I would like to discuss relates to culture and professional ethics. It is commonly accepted in Vietnamese families that parents do everything for their children, even planning their lives. In this case, the child is the only child in the family, and all of the parents' hope is placed on him. The medical staff in this case decided not to tell the truth because, according to their point of view: 'If we tell the parents about the real situation that the child will die – we would be taking the lives of the whole family.' Moreover, culturally they have learnt that it is not fair or right to destroy a whole family. It is a natural tendency that when people do not have full knowledge or understanding, the only thing they rely on for making decisions is what they have learnt from their culture and from their own feelings and experiences. The cultural factor is an important influence in this case.

In conclusion, when looking for any explanation for ethical decisions, it is useful to analyse the context and the cultural factors. What social workers can do in these situations is to share professional knowledge and skills in the ethical decision-making process and develop and deliver appropriate services.

Nguyen Thi Thai Lan is a social work lecturer at the University of Labour and Social Affairs, Hanoi, Vietnam, and a Ph.D. candidate, School of Social Sciences and International Studies, University of New South Wales, Australia.

Commentary 2

RICHARD HUGMAN

This is an interesting example of the challenge of thinking ethically about cross-cultural interactions in social work practice. In this situation the social work student has rightly, in my view, considered the question of the nature of the difference between her own values and those of the medical staff and teachers. Is this a difference between 'Dutch' and 'Vietnamese' values, or between someone who has been taught to think of her own professional role in breaking bad news and helping the person through this and those who do not have such knowledge or skills?

A further challenge is posed by the additional information from local people about how they see their own values, in that there is an expectation of not telling someone about the likely fatality of their condition. This implies that culturally 'being happy' is more valued than 'knowing the truth', especially when the person in question is a child. Western culture can be criticised from an Asian perspective as being overly focused on an individualistic understanding of rights, one that ignores other values such as happiness and harmony.

However, before we conclude that this is simply a matter of cultural difference, we must also note that the person in question is a child aged eight years old. It is also the case that the prognosis is not exact and has to be couched in terms of 'possibility'. The 'right to know' that might be more expected in a Western context would, I suggest, in this type of case attach to the parents and not necessarily to the child. That the parents have also not been told about the reality of Trung's condition is more surprising, even in an Asian cultural context. Vietnam has a modern constitution that includes the value of human rights and although the expression of these can often take different forms to those that might be seen in many Western countries, other factors must also be considered here. The health professionals do appear to have indicated that they are not well prepared for breaking bad news, which connects competence to other ethical issues, such as honesty and the rights of Trung and his family.

At the same time, there are other ethical approaches (in addition to those focusing on rights) that are relevant to understanding aspects of the 'good' in this situation. For example, the interaction between Trung and the physiotherapist closely resembles a description of the ethics of care in practice provided by Sevenhuijsen (1998: 1–2). It is attentive to Trung, in a way that is appropriate for an eight-year-old boy, and values qualities that he shows in his writing and drawing, and enables him to be responsive to this care. Trung's parents, similarly, are engaged in practical care for him that enables him to do as much of the normal activities that an eight-year-old might, allowing for his disability. This degree of care is also valued culturally, but as in other places is not always practised.

As professional social work develops in Vietnam it is likely that in the future there will be people within the social services system who can enable health colleagues to be more open with parents in this type of situation. The aim is for social workers to be able to provide the type of ongoing support to families facing these types of difficulties that will enable them to cope better with the realities that they face. When this happens, then a practical connection can be made between the ethics of rights and the ethics of care.

Reference

Sevenhuijsen, S. (1998) *Citizenship and the Ethics of Care: Feminist Considerations on Justice, Morality and Politics*, London: Routledge.

Richard Hugman is Professor of Social Work, University of New South Wales, Australia. Since 2004 he has worked with UNICEF Vietnam to advise the Vietnamese Government on the establishment of a social work profession in Vietnam.

Questions for discussion about Case 3.3

1 What does this case tell you about how the concept of 'rights' and, in particular, individuals' rights to information about themselves might be understood and valued in Vietnam and in Holland? How does this compare with your own country?

2 In your opinion, in what circumstances is it appropriate and ethically acceptable for a professional practitioner to withhold information about a patient's/service user's medical condition? How does this case compare with Case 4.2 about the young man taken off the waiting list for an organ transplant in Britain?

3 To what extent do you see this case exemplifying the distinction between the 'ethics of rights'/'ethics of justice' (exhibited by the Dutch student) and the 'ethics of care' (exhibited by Vietnamese physiotherapists) as discussed in the Introduction to Chapter 2? Is this distinction a helpful one, and what connection between the two approaches do you think can and should be made?

Case study 3.4

Case 3.4 Ethical issues in international social work research: a case from India

Introduction

On 26 December, 2004, an earthquake of magnitude 9.3 on the Richter scale triggered a tsunami in the Indian Ocean. The earthquake was felt widely along the coasts of India and while many people are believed to have died in the earthquake, most fatalities resulted from drowning caused by the seawater that gushed into the coastal areas. The earthquake, the tsunami and the events that followed will be long remembered as one of the worst human tragedies in history. Numerous studies on the 2004 tsunami and other natural and human-made disasters have found that there is a differential impact of disasters on affected populations, with a differential timeframe in their recovery. Many studies have documented this differential impact on marginalised communities such as poor people and excluded groups; their struggle to recover is slower than those with access to and control over resources. In South India, customs and norms adhere to a rigorous caste system that entraps marginalised Dalit people.[2] Prior to the tsunami, the livelihoods of many fishing folk were under stress, and the post-tsunami recovery and reconstruction efforts, in some cases, exacerbated their struggles and challenges.

Post-tsunami there was a massive international interest in the recovery efforts with unprecedented international humanitarian aid that flowed into the affected communities in many countries. Financial resources, trained personnel, humanitarian supplies and training became available in many communities. The distribution of these goods, services and materials took place through national governments, state districts and at the community level. However, there were many flaws in who received assistance and who did not, and whose needs were and were not met. Many marginalised fishing communities in South India faced not only social, economic and gendered impacts of the disaster, but also the struggle of trying to get their fair share of these relief materials.

The case

An international research team conducted a study on rebuilding lives post-tsunami by focusing on community narratives of affected fishing and non-fishing communities, Dalit communities, and indigenous tribal communities in the Nagapattinam district of Tamil Nadu, South India. At the planning stage, ethical questions were raised about who should be included in the study. This was an important consideration because if we had only gone by damage to property (boats and nets), or deaths (more

2 The term 'Dalit people' as used here refers to communities at the lowest level of the caste system in India. The caste system is a social stratification process in India. The Dalits were the outcasts in this stratification, always on the margins of society and constantly left out of the development process with no access to resources, as well as socially, economically and educationally marginalised. Religion played an important role in this marginalisation process, leaving them vulnerable to the higher castes.

among the fishing communities since they lived on the shore), we would have forgotten or not included the non-fishing, the Dalits, and the indigenous or tribal communities. An appreciation of the long-term direct and indirect impacts of a disaster like the tsunami, an understanding of how communities are linked and interdependent in the Indian context, a policy of taking the side of the marginalised and disadvantaged, as well as the strong values of social work embedded in the inclusion, helped us to decide on who should be included in the research sample.

The research team comprised social work researchers at five universities (Madras Christian College, Thompson Rivers University, Flinders University, University of South Australia and Appalachian State University) in four countries (India, Canada, Australia and the USA). The research team met in India to develop a memorandum of understanding that included values and principles for the duration of the research study. Yet it is complicated to coordinate places or venues to meet, to rely on communication by email and to understand emerging issues in gathering information from field research taking place in rural South India. The team relied extensively on the expertise and knowledge of Indian partners to develop research methods that were appropriate and sensitive to the context and culture. However, as community narratives emerged from the affected post-tsunami communities, it became apparent that a number of challenges and difficult issues needed to be addressed in terms of the long-term nature of the reconstruction, and the apparent discriminatory practices that impact the human rights of marginalised groups. In particular, there were ethical dilemmas that arose out of the research project.

As information about the troubles being faced by marginalised communities emerged, the researchers began to situate these concerns in the context of the study. It is important that all social work activity adheres to social work values and ethics, including social work research. Therefore, ethical issues came to the fore. If issues of violation of human rights, inequities, exploitation and denial of access to necessary resources for human dignity were identified, what did this mean for the social work researchers? Were they responsible for addressing the issues? Were they responsible for alerting others so that they may address them? What if other local service providers lacked capacity to do so? Were there ethical responsibilities to ensure support to these sources of resources?

Questions about for whom the research was being done, who the team was accountable to and who needed to take responsibility for the violation of marginalised people's human rights surfaced. For example, there were documented cases where higher caste groups and individuals used marginalised communities to gain more relief, but did not share the provisions or funding with these communities. The focus group discussions conducted documented the instances of differential intervention given to different marginalised groups post-tsunami. Households headed by single women, who were already marginalised socially, were further marginalised post-tsunami with no relief provided for them. Many excluded groups lacked compensation for loss of property, livestock or educational opportunities. Many affected communities still had a need for common community buildings and better sanitation, and food shortages were ongoing particularly for women and girls. During the study it was discovered that the housing provided for marginalised communities was poorer in quality and structure than that provided for the higher-caste fishing communities. Important research findings presented other ethical dilemmas. How does this information get disseminated in the field? How can we make this data available for communities? How could the researchers share the findings when power issues and human rights violations could present further risks for disadvantaged groups?

The research study was funded for a one-year period by the Social Sciences and Humanities Research Council of Canada, and was subsequently extended for a second year. The researchers complied with the Canadian Tri-Council funding guidelines on how the research funds could be spent in the course of the study. For example, it was not possible to develop an intervention after the needs of the communities emerged in the exploratory research study. If there were no restrictions the research team may have been able to explore interventions related to lobbying and advocacy roles for ensuring that the needs of marginalised groups were met. Other possibilities might include empowerment programmes for self-help groups, support for forming pressure/support groups in the communities, and training programmes for grass roots level NGOs working with these communities. The findings of the study demonstrated that as community members learned about their rights and their entitlements there was still a process needed to make the changes that were going to require a long-term effort. What responsibility does the research team have in engaging with affected communities to facilitate these changes? Is it the responsibility of the research team to facilitate these changes? What financial and human resources need to be acquired to address these issues? Or do we just remain silent spectators to the discriminatory practices?

As it became more and more obvious that the rights of these individuals and communities were being grossly violated, it became more difficult and more frustrating to stand by. But is it the responsibility of the researchers to change the circumstances of these people? If so, one must be sure to prevent cultural, religious and personal biases from determining the changes that are made. If not, what steps should be taken by the researchers to encourage those who are responsible to facilitate change?

Commentary 1

P. K. VISVESVARAN

Researchers drawn from five different universities situated in four different countries (Australia, Canada, the USA and India) have collaborated to conduct a study on the rehabilitation of the victims of the 2004 tsunami, the respondents being selected exclusively from the State of (coastal) Tamil Nadu in India. While undertaking the study, the researchers have come across instances of human rights violations, including denial of assistance to the needy, and some favoured few cornering the benefits. There were also acts of corruption on the part of those dispensing assistance.

Responses to the researchers' ethical questions

This dismaying experience has given rise, in the researchers' minds, to a number of ethical questions and dilemmas. In commenting on this case, I will offer responses to some of these questions (the questions raised by the researchers are given in italics).

What should violation of human rights mean for the researchers?

It cannot and should not mean the same thing to both the local researcher and the collaborators from abroad. For one thing, foreign investigators would have come to India, in all likelihood, as researchers and not as activists. It may not be ethical – it may even be illegal – to land here as scientists and don a different role (as change agents). The local researcher, however, faces a different kind of ethical dilemma. His/her professed role (working in a college) is that of educator. The cost of assuming a different role may be too heavy. Most colleges receive governmental aid, which would be stopped should they deviate from the stipulated path. Further, if college lecturers start playing an activist role, they will be exposing their students to threats and attacks from hostile forces and vested interests. Neither the parents of the students nor the government would take kindly to this prospect.

Were the researchers responsible for alerting others? What if the local service-providers lacked the capacity to act?

The researchers did have a responsibility to alert other key individuals and organisations about their findings. However, they could not take responsibility if local agencies did not have the resources or ability to take action. Capacity-building was not part of the researchers' mandate.

For whom was the research being done, and to whom were the researchers accountable?

The researchers were accountable only to the academic community – teachers and students – and to their own collective conscience.

How does this information get disseminated in the field?

English-medium newspapers in India would be most willing to publish such research findings (as the present commentator found, on more than one occasion). Also the researchers could undertake a trip to different colleges, especially in the South, to discuss their findings with the academic community.

Should the researchers remain silent spectators to discriminatory practices?

No, they should not remain silent. They could always lodge a complaint with the Human Rights Commissions in India, established under the Protection of Human Rights Act 1993.

Concluding remarks

Almost all Indian colleges and their departments lack the moral authority to fight inequity elsewhere, since they themselves practise it all the time. Moreover, gross discrimination is built into governmental policies and budget allocation practices. For example, in India, a state government spends 50 per cent of its revenue on just two per cent of its population, namely the government servants. This could be one of the reasons for the corrupt practices we see at lower levels.

Finally, it should be stated here that if the tsunami has brought to light discriminatory practices and human rights violations in India, they should not be viewed as a sudden or isolated development that could be nipped in the bud. They may only be symptomatic of anomalies that pervade the entire social fabric. Outsiders could do little about them, and insiders themselves can only acquaint all right-thinking and service-minded people with the existing realities. Changes will come only in the long run.

P. K. Visvesvaran, Master of Philosophy in Social Work, served as a faculty member at the Madras School of Social Work, India, for 32 years from 1970 until retirement in 2002. Articles on professional topics have been published in the *Indian Journal of Social Work* and the *Journal of School Social Work*. He currently gives guest lectures in several colleges, including the Madras Christian College, Tambaram.

Commentary 2

WENDY BOWLES AND MARGARET ALSTON

The issue

This case raises complex ethical questions relating to research conducted by an international team on the impact of disaster relief efforts in post-tsunami Southern India. The research study focused on narratives about how lives were being rebuilt. It draws attention to the increased vulnerability of the households headed by single women, the Dalit communities and indigenous tribal communities not based on fishing, but nonetheless affected by the tsunami. It gives an account of how the researchers became aware that aid was not reaching the most vulnerable even when sourced in their name.

This raises significant ethical issues for the researchers as to whether they should intervene and if so in what way. It is important to acknowledge that the kinds of issues raised in this case are not confined to South India, and have been raised by researchers and relief workers across the global South when engaging in post-disaster work (see, for example, Terry 2009). Responses to disasters on the scale of the 2004 tsunami bring their own significant impacts to social structures in the countries affected. For example, Pandya (2006) argues that in post-tsunami Aceh and Nias, the relatively huge amount of resources flooding the region through non-governmental organisations (NGOs) has meant that various players in the private sector now wield power and authority that was previously only held by the state. Pandya (ibid.: 307) comments: 'In the process, private authority has become a legitimate but unaccountable player in poor countries.'

In this case at least five key stakeholder groups can be identified, all with their own ethical bases from which they operate and which most likely also encompass divisions and conflict. The most obvious stakeholder, with a powerful voice in the situation, is the research funding body, the Social Sciences and Humanities Research Council of Canada. The case states that the Council's guidelines prohibit spending research funds making interventions after the needs of the communities are identified in the exploratory research study – a prohibition with which the researchers complied.

The next stakeholder group, comprising social work researchers in five universities from India, Canada, Australia and the USA, would have their own university research ethics principles to which they are bound. In addition, as emphasised in the case, the researchers felt obliged to meet their ethical obligations as social workers, with their commitment to social justice and human rights (IFSW and IASSW 2000, 2004). The case outlines how these values influence the nature of the research question and the research design, including the decision to include marginalised and disadvantaged groups. However, even within the social work research team of five universities, it is by no means certain that team members held shared understandings of social work values. For example, given the current debate within international social work about whether the ethical principles expressed in the IFSW and IASSW statement are actually 'professional imperialism' imposed by global Northern social work on social work in the global South (see for example Banks 2008; Hugman 2008, 2010), there may well have been divisions within the team about the ethical obligations of the researchers in relation to whether and how they should intervene.

The third stakeholder group, and quite an influential one in terms of what data is recorded, is the Indian partners on whom the researchers are relying in order to develop culturally appropriate and sensitive research methods. It is not clear whether they are also social workers.

The fourth group to be considered is the NGOs and other aid organisations that were providing the relief efforts and whose outcomes were being evaluated by the research team. This group encompasses both local and international organisations, private and public, with their own ethical codes and imperatives, and differing levels of power and influence, as noted above.

The fifth group, which was the direct focus of the research study, includes the various community groups whose narratives were being collected and analysed to determine the effects of the post-disaster relief efforts.

As the authors of the case study point out, a major difficulty in addressing this question is that the accountability of the research project was not clear from the start. There are at least four other groups to whom the researchers may have been accountable, but it is not clear whether this was part of the project or not. The discussion at the end of the case about empowering self-help groups, training grass roots NGOs and working with community members to make long-term changes once rights and entitlements were made clear, implies some accountability to the NGOs and the communities being researched, as well as to the Canadian funding body.

Ethical issues

The case study concludes with an ethical question that is raised by many kinds of research both within countries and in international contexts. This is: When researchers become aware of violations of human rights or other kinds of ethical breaches, what are their obligations? Should they intervene or not? If so, in what capacity? The authors of the case add a precaution that 'one must be sure to prevent cultural, religious and personal biases from determining the changes that are made'. Several ethical issues and questions arise from the case, including the following:

- Does violation of human rights 'trump' the obligation from the Canadian Tri-Council guidelines not to use research funds to intervene and is this actually possible, if research findings are being reported to various stakeholder groups?
- Could the researchers act in parallel with the research process, as social workers with particular knowledge, rather than researchers? Or could action take place after the project and with other funds? In which case, the question becomes how do the researchers intervene without being imperialist?
- It would seem impossible to prevent cultural and religious biases as the authors advocate. Indeed, this seems to presuppose that there is only one cultural stance within the South Indian context, and we know this is not the case. There are many cultural and racial groups involved, so we are in a culturally plural context for a start. Even within one group there is often division and debate and different voices. The researchers' opinions may align with one side or another and they must determine how to use their power responsibly, perhaps to ensure that all people's needs are met. Thus it would seem appropriate to undertake respectful conversations about the research outcomes and implications with the key stakeholders.
- Within this complex situation it is important that the researchers themselves acknowledge the debate within international social work about professional imperialism.

As Australian social work researchers, our experience is that these kinds of ethical questions arise regularly in social work research, within national as well as international contexts. Possibly this is partly due to the nature of social work research, which so often involves situations of disadvantage and oppression, fuelled by social work's ethical imperatives to enhance human rights and well-being and social justice, as argued in the case study.

Indeed, with the rise of service user movements, and action research approaches in which research participants are partners, the boundaries between research and social action are no longer as clear as the prohibition by the Canadian Tri-Council implies. While hindsight is powerful, it may be useful for social work researchers to consider writing some form of action into future research designs from the beginning. For example, some forms of action research employ a reflective cycle involving changes within whatever is being researched in response to the findings, as one of the desired research outcomes. Similarly, researchers may work with reference groups including representatives of research participants (such as Aboriginal and Torres Strait Islander communities, or disability groups), who are responsible for considering the results and have a strong voice in the recommendations being made to government or policy makers.

The ethical issues in this case are complex. In summary, we would argue that when social workers know that the rights of vulnerable people are being exploited they cannot stand idly by and do nothing. The question becomes not if action should taken but when and how.

References

Banks, S. (2008) 'Critical commentary: social work ethics', *British Journal of Social Work*, 38(6):1238–1249.

Hugman, R. (2008) 'Ethics in a world of difference', *Ethics and Social Welfare*, 2(2): 118–132.

Hugman, R. (2010) *Understanding International Social Work: A Critical Analysis*, Basingstoke: Palgrave Macmillan.

Ife, J. (2008) *Human Rights in Social Work: Towards Rights-Based Practice*, revised edition, Port Melbourne, VIC: Cambridge University Press.

International Federation of Social Workers (IFSW) and International Association of Schools of Social Work (IASSW) (2000) *Definition of Social Work*, Berne: IFSW and IASSW (available at www.ifsw.org/f38000138. html).

International Federation of Social Workers (IFSW) and International Association of Schools of Social Work (IASSW) (2004) *Ethics in Social Work: Statement of Principles*, Berne: IFSW and IASSW.

Pandya, C. (2006) 'Private authority and disaster relief: the cases of post-tsunami Aceh and Nias', *Critical Asian Studies*, 38(2): 298–308.

Terry, G. (2009) 'No climate justice without gender justice: an overview of the issues', *Gender and Development*, 17(1): 5–18.

Wendy Bowles is Associate Professor of Social Work and Human Services in the School of Humanities and Social Sciences at Charles Sturt University, Wagga Wagga, NSW, Australia.

Margaret Alston, OAM, is Professor of Social Work and Head of Department at Monash University, Melbourne, Australia.

Questions for discussion about Case 3.4

1 What do you think are the responsibilities of social work researchers who witness or uncover instances of injustice, oppression or deception? What difference does it make if the researchers are from another country?

2 Are you aware of any codes of ethics for researchers in social sciences and/or social work in your country or internationally? Do they offer any guidance that might be relevant to this case?

3 The two commentaries on this case offer some answers to the questions raised by the researchers and give recommendations for action. To what extent are the perspectives offered by the commentators complementary or in conflict?

4 | Being fair

Introduction

FREDERIC REAMER

The centrality of fairness in social work

Throughout the profession's history, social workers have been preoccupied with fairness, a complex concept that is ordinarily associated with qualities of justice, equity, impartiality, neutrality and the absence of discrimination and bias. Since the late nineteenth century, when social work was formally inaugurated in Europe and the United States, the concept of fairness has been prominent in the profession. Social workers' earliest concern about fairness focused especially on the problem of increasing poverty, and inequity in the distribution of wealth. For many years social workers addressed the nagging problems of inadequate housing, health care, and income, particularly the impact of persistent unfairness in the allocation of social and economic resources and wealth. Over time, social workers (particularly in the global North) began to focus more narrowly on mental health and behavioural challenges posed by individual clients and families, many of which are the by-products of daunting discrimination, oppression, exploitation and other manifestations of unfairness in society (Trattner 1999).

Social work's enduring and admirable preoccupation with issues of fairness is particularly evident in codes of ethics adopted throughout the world. For example, the statement of the International Federation of Social

Workers and International Association of Schools of Social Work (2004), *Ethics in Social Work, Statement of Principles*, features several principles pertaining directly to issues of fairness, particularly related to confronting negative discrimination, recognising diversity, distributing resources equitably and challenging unjust policies and practices. The British Association of Social Workers' (2002) *Code of Ethics* includes multiple references to issues of fairness, especially related to the fair and equitable distribution of resources, fair access to public services and benefits, equal treatment and protection under the law, and non-discrimination. The Canadian Association of Social Workers' *Code of Ethics* (2005) states that 'social workers promote social fairness and the equitable distribution of resources', and the USA's National Association of Social Workers' *Code of Ethics* (2008) features several core principles related to social justice, non-discrimination and fairness in the allocation of social and economic resources.

The historical and philosophical roots of fairness

The concepts of fairness and justice have ancient historical and philosophical origins (Williams 1993). Plato's *Republic* begins with the question, 'What is justice?' In his *Politics*, Aristotle argues that justice entails treating equals equally and unequals unequally. Aristotle highlights the importance of non-arbitrary, consistent treatment of people according to morally relevant attributes. In the seventeenth century the English philosopher John Locke (1690) explored fairness and social justice issues in his *Second Treatise of Civil Government*, and Karl Marx (1848) stirred considerable debate about distributive justice in his nineteenth-century classic published with Engels, the *Communist Manifesto*.

Contemporary moral philosophers have done much to sustain focus on issues of fairness. For example, since its publication John Rawls' (1971) *A Theory of Justice* has shaped countless discussions of fairness in modern society, as has Robert Nozick's (1974) publication, *Anarchy, State and Utopia*.

Prominent philosophical commentaries on fairness focus on a number of key moral concepts that are applicable to the kinds of ethical challenges that social workers encounter and that are featured in this chapter's case studies.

Theoretical schools of thought

Classic discussions of ethics and moral philosophy typically compare and contrast deontological and teleological perspectives (Rachels 2002). These contrasting schools of thought have profoundly different implications for fairness issues that arise in social work (Dolgoff, Loewenberg and Harrington 2008, Reamer 2006, Timms 1983). Deontological theories (from the Greek *deontos*, 'of the obligatory') are those that claim that certain actions are inherently right or wrong, or good or bad, without regard for their consequences. Thus a deontologist – the best known is Immanuel Kant, the eighteenth-century German philosopher – might argue that people ought to have fully equal access to scarce or limited social resources as a matter of inherent fairness, even if an unequal distribution would promote more social and economic good in the long run. For Kant (1797), certain acts are morally right or fair if they are consistent with his 'categorical imperative', by which he meant that one should act in a certain fashion only if one can, at the same time, assert that it should become a universal law. For deontologists, rules, rights and principles are inviolable. Similarly, a deontologist might argue that a law should always be obeyed, regardless of the consequences. That is, the ends do not necessarily justify the means, particularly if they require violating an inherent right. Hence a deontologist might claim that in Case 4.1 the social worker had a fundamental duty to obey Japanese law and agency policy that prohibits offering public assistance to foreigners. Similarly, a deontologist might argue that the young patient in Case 4.2 had a fundamental right to the truth about his health condition and the fact that he had been removed from the waiting list for a transplant; lying to the patient would violate a sacred moral principle and would not be justifiable as a means to some other end (for example, to protect the patient from emotional harm).

In contrast, teleological theories (from the Greek *teleios*, 'brought to its end or purpose') take a different approach to ethical choices. From this point of view, the rightness of any moral choice is determined by the goodness of its consequences. Teleologists think that it is naïve to make ethical choices without weighing potential consequences. To do otherwise is to engage in what the moral philosopher Smart (1971) referred to as 'rule worship'. Therefore, from this perspective (sometimes known as consequentialism), the responsible strategy entails an attempt to forecast the outcomes of various courses of action. For instance, what are the benefits and harms involved in lying to or withholding information from a client, interfering with a client's right to self-determination, or obeying an unjust law? In Case 4.1, for example, the social worker might argue that the harm caused by violating Japanese law and agency policy would be outweighed by the good that would result from offering public assistance to the mother and her child. In Case 4.3 the social worker would need to weigh the likely benefits and harms if the social worker were to help his young client pursue her dream of staying in school, as opposed to acceding to the gypsy community's cultural norms.

The best-known school of teleological thought is utilitarianism, which holds that an action is morally right if it promotes the maximum good. According to the classic form of utilitarianism – as originally formulated by the English philosophers Jeremy Bentham (1789) in the eighteenth century and John Stuart Mill (1863) in the nineteenth century – when faced with conflicting duties one should do that which will produce the greatest good (positive utilitarianism) or minimise harm (negative utilitarianism). When making decisions about fairness, social workers should enter into a calculus that weighs all anticipated benefits and costs. In Case 4.4, for example, the social worker would weigh the potential benefits and harms if she permits the client (a gay man) to adopt a child in a culture that has little tolerance for homosexuality. The calculus would consider the impact of the decision on the child, client, social worker, agency and broader society.

One form of utilitarianism that is particular germane to discussions of fairness is known as 'good-aggregative utilitarianism', according to which the fairest action is that which promotes the greatest total or aggregate good. Another theory is 'locus-aggregative utilitarianism', according to which the fairest action is that which promotes the greatest good for the greatest number, considering not only the total quantity of goods produced but also the number of people to whom the goods are distributed (Gewirth 1978). The distinction between these two forms of utilitarianism is important in social work when practitioners decide how to allocate limited resources, such as agency funds, staffers' time and social services.

Another philosophical distinction that is important in social work is between act and rule utilitarianism. According to act utilitarianism, the rightness of an action is determined by the goodness of the consequences in that individual case, or by that particular act. In Case 4.3, for instance, the social worker would weigh the potential benefits and harms in this one case involving the young gypsy girl who wants to remain in school. How would she be affected if the social worker respected her wishes and helped her stay in school? How might she be harmed? What are the possible benefits and harms to the family, the local gypsy community, the broader community and the social worker?

By contrast, rule utilitarianism takes into account the long-term consequences likely to result if one generalises from the case at hand and treats it as a precedent. What are the likely benefits and harms in the long run if the actions the social worker takes in the case are treated as a precedent for future comparable cases? If all similarly situated clients are treated in the same way, what impact would this have on the clients themselves, the professionals and the broader community? For instance, in Case 4.1 the rule utilitarian perspective would require one to consider the long-term impact if the social worker's decision to violate Japanese law and agency policy were treated as a precedent and generalised to all comparable cases.

Moral absolutism and relativism

Social workers have embraced these diverse perspectives, sometimes more implicitly than explicitly, in their efforts to promote fairness. Some practitioners, reflecting the philosophical perspective known as cognitivism, believe that it is possible to establish universal principles and objective criteria upon which to base ethical judgements about fairness. This view is also known as absolutism. For instance, based on this view the social worker in Case 4.4 would not factor into her ethical decision the unique cultural norms in the Turkish community; rather, the social worker would claim that there are universal ethical standards, regardless of local culture, that should be applied in this case, such as the universal principle of non-discrimination. Others – known as relativists or non-cognitivists – argue instead that ethical standards are not fixed or immutable but, rather, depend on cultural beliefs, political values, contemporary norms and moral standards, and other contextual considerations. In Case 4.3, according to relativism, the social worker would take into consideration the gypsy community's cultural beliefs related to the role of women in society, schooling and marriage norms.

Prominent fairness themes in social work

The cases in this chapter demonstrate that issues of fairness arise in clinical social work and in social work that involves social advocacy, policy formulation and implementation and community organising. In clinical social work, compelling issues of fairness arise when social workers decide whether they must always be truthful with clients or are permitted, morally, to lie to or deceive clients (see Case 4.2). Clinical social workers also make judgements about fairness when they decide whether they are morally obligated to obey all rules, laws, and policies related to their clients (see Case 4.1), and whether it is ever permissible to discriminate against a client on the basis of race, ethnicity, national origin, colour, sex, sexual orientation, gender identity or expression, age, marital status, political belief, religion, immigration status, or mental or physical disability (see Cases 4.1, 4.3 and 4.4).

By contrast, social workers involved in administration, advocacy and social policy must make judgements about the fair and just allocation of social, organisational and economic resources, particularly when they are in short supply. For example, the professionals involved in Case 4.2 had to establish criteria and procedures to guide the allocation of scarce organs for transplantation, just as agency administrators and political officials must often establish mechanisms to distribute limited funds. Further, social workers who are in administrative, advocacy and policy positions must be cognisant of principles of fairness that pertain to various forms of discrimination, as in Case 4.1 about the Filipino woman classed as an illegal immigrant in Japan.

Pursuing fairness in social work

One of social work's principal virtues is its enduring concern about matters of fairness. Unique among the ethical frameworks of the various human service professions, prominent social work codes of ethics throughout the world consistently highlight the central importance of fairness, justice, equity, impartiality, neutrality and non-discrimination. Although reasonable minds can differ about the strengths and limitations of different theoretical approaches to fairness, social workers agree that the pursuit of fairness is among the most compelling elements of social work's mission. It is this unique preoccupation that distinguishes social work as a noble profession.

References

Bentham, J. (1789) [1948 edition] *An Introduction to the Principles of Morals and Legislation*, New York: Hafner.

British Association of Social Workers (2002) *The Code of Ethics for Social Work*, Birmingham: BASW.

Canadian Association of Social Workers (CASW) (2005) *Code of Ethics*, Ottawa: CASW.

Dolgoff, R., Loewenberg, F. and Harrington, D. (2008) *Ethical Decisions for Social Work Practice*, 8th edition, Belmont, CA: Brooks Cole.

Gewirth, A. (1978) *Reason and Morality*, Chicago: University of Chicago Press.

International Federation of Social Workers and International Association of Schools of Social Work (2004) *Ethics in Social Work, Statement of Principles*, IFSW and IASSW, Berne (available at: www.ifsw.org).

Kant, I. (1797) [1959 edition] *Foundations of the Metaphysics of Morals*, translated by. L. W. Beck, New York: Liberal Arts Press.

Locke, J. (1690) [1978 edition] *Second Treatise of Civil Government*, Grand Rapids, MI: W. B. Eerdsman.

Marx, K. and Engels, F. (1848) [1967 edition] *Communist Manifesto*, New York: Penguin.

Mill, J. (1863) [1957 edition] *Utilitarianism*, Indianapolis: Bobbs-Merrill.

National Association of Social Workers (2008) *Code of Ethics*, Washington: NASW.

Nozick, R. (1974) *Anarchy, State and Utopia*, Blackwell: Oxford.

Rachels, J. (2002) *Elements of Moral Philosophy*, 4th edition, Boston: McGraw-Hill.

Rawls, J. (1971) *A Theory of Justice*, Cambridge, MA: The Belknap Press of Harvard University Press.

Reamer, F. (2006) *Social Work Values and Ethics*, 3rd edition, New York: Columbia University Press.

Smart, J. (1971) 'Extreme and restricted utilitarianism', in S. Gorovitz (ed.) *Mill: Utilitarianism*, Indianapolis: Bobbs-Merrill.

Timms, N. (1983) *Social Work Values: An Enquiry*, London: Routledge and Kegan Paul.

Trattner, W. (1999) *From Poor Law to Welfare State*, 6th edition, New York: Free Press.

Williams, B. (1993) *Morality: An Introduction to Ethics*, Cambridge: Cambridge University Press.

Case study 4.1

Case 4.1 Dilemmas in working with an illegal migrant: a case from Japan

Introduction

This case has been written by a social worker in Japan who was working in a public welfare office. In Japan, every prefecture and city has an obligation to establish a public welfare office. These offices generally provide social services (income benefits and personal social services) for those who need social welfare. Many officers working in the public welfare offices have not necessarily been trained and qualified as social workers.

The case

This case relates to the time about 15 years ago when I was a young state social worker working in the public welfare office of a Japanese city. I was a qualified social worker, with higher education training. I was working as a welfare officer who was in charge of public assistance to the poor whose income was below the national poverty line.

One day another officer discovered a woman from the Philippines and her child who had escaped from another area. They were being sheltered by a charity organisation when I met them. The charity told me that this woman and her child needed income security and other related assistance from the state, as their income level was below the national poverty line.

I interviewed the woman about her life history and why she had fallen into poverty. This revealed that she was a migrant worker from the Philippines. She had come to Japan for the purpose of collecting money to maintain her own family, which was living in the Philippines. She was probably around 30 years old (she looked younger) and she came to Japan to work as a dancer in a hot spring resort in the countryside. She did not have a legal 'work visa' and lived with her boyfriend, who was a Japanese cook in the same workplace. After a year, she had a daughter with him. However, a few years later her boyfriend suddenly disappeared and left her on her own with her daughter. She found she was not able to do her work properly and care for her child at the same time. So she ran away from her workplace.

I asked her some questions in the interview: 'So, you are not legally married to your Japanese boyfriend?' She confirmed that she was not legally married. I said to her, 'Did you register your child's birth with the town office?' She said to me, 'No.' This state of affairs was typical for illegal migrants. Yet she and her child needed social work service because of their situation. More importantly, her child was obviously of mixed parentage, but this child only spoke the Japanese language (she did not understand English). Her daughter looked as though she was three or four years old.

If the woman had married her boyfriend legally, her legal position would be regarded as 'non-problematic'. But she was not married. This was a big concern and caused a dilemma for me. As a social worker, I wanted to try to protect her and her child and to help them reorganise their lives. I thought they also had a human right to live continuously in Japan. But there was a big barrier in front of me: the problem of 'nationality'. Foreigners are not eligible for public assistance and as a migrant her status was not recognised in law, as she was not legally married to her Japanese boyfriend.

As a social worker and a public officer, what should I do? I had a dilemma. If I set them free from my own office, they would probably be free from the enslavement of legal problems (because she had a possibility to marry another Japanese man and to live as a Japanese citizen from the legal point of view). But the mother and daughter could not be given social services from the state. Certainly she did not know why social services from the state did not respond quickly to foreigners. She was a good citizen who was keen to live in Japan with her child. Nevertheless, her wish was not granted.

I tried to take some actions with my colleagues by means of looking for foster care, but the Ministry of Welfare issued a circular to the public welfare offices saying that it was against the law to offer public assistance to foreigners. While we were trying to make efforts, the chief officer in my welfare office reported this case to the police, because of the migration issues. In the end, the woman and her child were detained by the police and the government immigration office on the grounds that she was in violation of migration laws. Her child (who was obviously half Japanese) was also sent back home with her mother, in spite of the fact that the child was not able to speak English.

As an ethical social worker, I would like to have taken more action to protect her human rights, but at the same time I was a civil servant with a legal obligation to uphold the civil law. My supervisor also told me that if the woman had married legally this problem would not have happened. However, I did not agree with the result of the case in terms of social work ethics (social justice and human rights).

Commentary 1

AKIRA NAMAE

Being called a 'social worker' does not always mean the work promotes social justice. This case shows a dilemma between so-called 'social work' and social justice. If justice was regarded simply as conforming to the law, as long as civil servants follow the law they could be regarded as fulfilling their roles legally. However, the social worker in this case was unable to agree with this kind of legal treatment, as he saw this case in terms of social work ethics based on the principles of social justice and human rights. This case exemplifies the difficulties faced by social workers working in public welfare offices in Japan, where the prevailing attitudes towards the poor in general are punitive and authoritarian.

Who is a criminal and who is a victim?

In this case, the illegal status of the Filipino mother was regarded as the main problem. Is this true? Certainly her visa was invalid and she was an illegal migrant. She was probably not aware of her visa status. However, we need to review this case from the viewpoint of the child. The child's birth and details of her parents had not been registered. Was her mother solely responsible for her birth? Her father seems to have been forgotten by the Japanese civil servants. He is one of the criminals in this case as he abandoned his responsibility to register and bring up his child. The girl is a victim. Did the Japanese civil servants know this? Or did they accept the crime and blame only the mother? Justice might involve simply focusing on a law; however, *social* justice does not always consist of one law and one criminal. After the mother and child went back to the Philippines it would become very difficult to look for the girl's father and make him accept that he was her father. If we were cynical, we might wonder whether he was a good friend of the civil servants (which might explain their decision to ignore his role in this case). We should certainly ask whether the attitude of the civil servants was fair to the girl in terms of social work ethics, based on principles of social justice and human rights.

Do illegal migrants or inhabitants have no human rights?

According to Japanese law about nationality, a baby takes its father's nationality. Therefore, in this case, as long as the civil servants could not deny the fact legally, they could not have deprived the girl of her nationality. In a sense, civil servants must receive instructions from their managers, as long as legal instructions conform to the law. If the girl's parent who came to the office had been her father, and if he insisted he was her father, he would have been asked to prove the truth of the claimed father-daughter relationship by means of a DNA test.

In this case we can see how gender and ethnic prejudice can easily result in the exclusion of illegal migrants from the realm of justice. However, the principles of social justice and human rights are not negotiable items that can be distributed to some and not others. The exclusion of certain people from these rights does not make for a socially just society, but rather an exclusive organisation or faction. A dilemma is often a starting point, rather than a conclusion, for social work. The principles of social justice and human rights are not given by society; rather the process of taking action for the principles yields our ethics and our society.

Akira Namae is Professor of Politics, Nihon Fukushi University, Japan.

Commentary 2

SHIMON E. SPIRO

Labour force migration has become a universal phenomenon. In many industrialised countries labour migrants are now a large part of the work-force. In most countries many of the labour migrants are 'illegal', either because they entered the country illegally, or because of changes in their employment or marital status. The stance of the social work profession towards 'illegal' immigrants and the application of social work ethics to this group are issues which have not been adequately addressed. This case provides an opportunity to explore some of these issues.

Codes of ethics, issued by social workers' associations all over the world, usually open with a statement requiring social workers to 'uphold each person's physical, psychological, emotional and spiritual integrity and well-being' (IFSW and IASSW 2004). Codes of ethics usually do not make exclusions. 'Each person' includes illegal migrants and their children. On the other hand, governments do make exclusions, and illegal migrants (in some cases even legal labour migrants) are often treated as non-persons. When oppressed or exploited they have no recourse to justice; when in need they are not eligible for assistance. Their children often do not legally exist, since their hunted parents are wary of registering births. Children who do not exist do not get the most basic services, such as inoculations, medical attention or education.

Japan, like almost all other countries (140 of them), signed and ratified the United Nations Convention on the Rights of the Child (1989). The countries that signed the convention committed themselves to 'ensure the rights of each child within their jurisdiction' (ibid.: article 2). By sign-ing the convention they agreed that 'in all actions concerning children, whether undertaken by private or public social welfare institutions, courts of law, administrative authorities or legislative bodies, the best interests of the child shall be a primary consideration' (ibid.: article 3). The con-vention proceeds to list the rights of children to education, health care and an adequate standard of living. It also states the right of the child to be cared for by both parents, irrespective of their marital status.

One can easily sympathise with the sense of helplessness expressed by the social worker who wrote the case. At the time she (or he) was young, inexperienced and powerless. However, the behaviour of the agency was patently unethical. Enforcing immigration laws is the business of the police and the courts, not of social welfare agencies, even if they are part of a municipal bureaucracy. It is their business, and the obligation of their employees, to ensure the well-being of persons in need, whatever their legal status. In this specific case there can be no doubt about the right of the child for health services, education and income support (either from the state or from the abandoning father), and the need of the mother for legal aid and material support.

The IFSW and IASSW (2004) code of ethics states that social workers have an obligation to 'challenge unjust policies and practices', and 'to work towards an inclusive society'. An application of these principles would require the author of the case, and her/his colleagues, to engage in efforts to change the policies and practices of the agency. Furthermore, social workers anywhere should engage in efforts to challenge national policies pertaining to 'illegal' migrants in general, with specific reference to children of mixed parentage. Such actions may not have helped the client discussed in this case, but might prevent similar injustices in the future.

It goes without saying that all aspects of professional ethics apply to all actual and potential clients of social workers and their agencies. However, since 'illegal' labour migration has become such a widespread phenomenon, a revision of national and international codes of ethics may be in order, so that they are explicit about the ethical obligations of professionals towards persons who, for whatever reason, have been legally excluded from society.

References

International Federation of Social Workers and International Association of Schools of Social Work (2004) *Ethics in Social Work, Statement of Principles*, IFSW and IASSW, www.ifsw.org, accessed November 2010.
United Nations (1989) *Convention on the Rights of the Child*, www.ohchr.org, accessed November 2010.

Shimon E. Spiro, Ph.D., is Associate Professor of Social Work and Sociology (retired), Tel Aviv University, Tel Aviv, Israel.

Questions for discussion about Case 4.1

1 Do you think the Filipino woman and her child were treated fairly by the Japanese authorities? How would you justify your answer with reference to either ethical theories or professional codes of ethics?

2 Do you think the distinction between legal justice and social justice is a useful one? What are the implications of this distinction for social workers?

3 If social workers witness or are party to unfair treatment of service users, or the implementation of unfair laws, what action do you think they can or should take? How easy do you think it would be for the social worker in this case, working in a public welfare office where the attitudes towards the poor are generally punitive, to resist the prevailing norms and culture?

Case study 4.2

Case 4.2 A young man waiting for a transplant: dilemmas for a hospital-based social worker in Britain

Introduction

This case is about a social worker based in a specialist hospital in Britain, and concerns a young person needing a heart and lung transplant. In Britain, hospital social workers are usually managed by local authority adult or children's services departments, which are located outside of the hospital itself. Many social workers work in multidisciplinary teams, which include medical and nursing staff, physiotherapists, occupational therapists and teaching staff. The role of medical consultants in the teams varies depending on the setting, the extent to which collaborative working has developed and the particular issue in question – which may not be a purely medical one. A national protocol for heart and lung transplants has been in place since 2002.[1] This sets out the criteria for assessing and prioritising patients for organ donation, offers clear grounds where organs can be refused and recommends that decisions are made following consideration by the whole team caring for individual patients.

1 NHS Blood and Transplant Cardiothoracic Advisory Group (2002, revised 2009) *National Protocol for Assessment of CardiothoracicTransplant Patients*, www. organdonation.nhs.uk/ukt/about_transplants/organ_allocation/cardiothoracic/nati onal_protocols_and_standards/protocols_and_standards/assessment_of_cardiothor acic_patients.pdf

In Britain, more people need transplanted organs than there are organs available. All patients requiring donor organs are registered by their medical consultant on the National Transplant Database. When donor organs become available, they are allocated to the best matched patient or most appropriate transplant centre (transplants take place in a few specialist centres in Britain). The exact arrangements depend on the organs donated. Donor organs are 'matched' to potential patients using criteria such as: compatibility (factors such as blood group can be relevant here); age of recipient; location of organs and potential recipient; as well as the urgency of the need for transplant.

The case

The social worker was a 35-year-old woman who had worked for eight years with adults and children affected by life-threatening illness. She had worked at this specialist hospital for five years. The hospital was also a transplant centre. Most of the social worker's caseload comprised young adults and teenagers with life-threatening heart and lung disease. As well as arranging for local support services for patients when they left hospital, she also worked with individuals, couples and families who wished to look at the emotional, practical and other aspects of life-threatening and often end-stage illness. Many patients were on the national waiting list for heart and/or heart and lung transplants, which could significantly extend their lifespan and dramatically improve their quality of life.

The young people on the waiting list were often desperate for a chance to be given donor organs, understanding that in order to be considered for this procedure, they had to be so seriously ill that there was no other option.

The social worker attended the ward round every week – a meeting chaired by the medical consultant and attended by about 15 other professionals. On this particular occasion, there was, as usual, a number of interesting discussions involving different perspectives from everyone in the large multi-professional team. This week the physiotherapist led a discussion about a 19-year-old man on the waiting list for a heart and lung transplant. She outlined how his health had deteriorated considerably over the past fortnight, and that his prognosis was now likely to be months at best.

The social worker had been working with this young man and his family for several months, trying to enable him to stay out of hospital as much as possible. The whole multi-professional team had worked with this young man and his family for many years – in the consultant's case, since his birth. Two years previously, his younger brother had died from the same condition. Hospital staff, as well as the man and his family, were anxious that donor organs would soon become available.

This week's ward round discussion took a difficult turn when the team came to focus on the young man in question. It was the occupational therapist who voiced what many colleagues had been thinking privately – that this young person was now not well enough to have a transplant, even if organs did become available. He would be unlikely to survive the surgery and would probably only live for a few months if he did survive. Therefore, she suggested, he should be removed from the transplant waiting list. In the unlikely event of his health improving in a few months, he could then be put back on the list.

This was a very painful decision for the team to make, but everyone came to the difficult realisation that it would be unethical to use precious donor organs in a situation so precarious, and where effectively they would be wasted. The discussion now moved on to consider how this information was going to be passed on to the young man and his family. After a lengthy discussion, the team came to the view that the young man should not be told that he was no longer on the transplant waiting list. Neither should his parents be informed. The social worker put forward her view that the young man had a right to know that his prognosis was so poor and that he was likely to die in a matter of months. She argued that however difficult it was to have this kind of conversation with the young man and his family, it was wrong to avoid being truthful and it was denying opportunities for the family to talk and plan together for the future.

The ward nurses took a different view. They suggested that it was not necessary to spell out to the young man that he was very sick, and that when the time came he and his family would probably ask questions about his prognosis and approaching death. It would be cruel, they said, to rob him of any kind of hope and to emphasise that his one chance of a better quality and length of life was no longer available. Not telling him the truth was not the same as deliberately lying, they argued.

The consultant asked the team what they thought she should do if the young man or his parents asked her directly whether or not he was still on the transplant waiting list. She reminded her colleagues that only a few months previously, a teenager with the same condition as this young man had committed suicide in the hospital. This teenager had remained on the waiting list but had lost hope of ever getting donor organs. She had become progressively weaker, barely able to walk or to move about without portable oxygen. This was something which was still deeply affecting the whole team, especially the nurses who had witnessed the incident. The consultant argued that removing hope for this young man and his family could have similarly devastating consequences. Of course, she said, the team had a duty to think about the young man – his rights, their duties, the consequences of lying or telling the truth. But they should also think about this ethical dilemma in the context of the hospital team and other patients and families. This was about more than this one individual.

The social worker was not happy with the team's consensus that they would not tell the young man that he had been removed from the waiting list. There was a shared view that the young man was unlikely to consider that he was no longer on the list, because such a possibility was not discussed with patients. The team believed that patients assumed that once they were on the list, they remained on it until they (hopefully) received their transplant. The social worker argued that she did not think there was much difference between withholding the truth or deliberately lying in this case. Privately, however, she was relieved that neither the young man nor his family asked her or any of the team any direct questions about this.

Afterwards

Some two months later the young man's health deteriorated sharply. Having had friends and his own brother die of the same condition, he knew that he too was dying. He was able to share this knowledge and his final few weeks with his parents, dying at home and talking openly about the fact that there was no longer any possibility of his body being able to use donor organs, as he was too sick.

Commentary 1

TAMARA CATCHPOLE HORSBURGH AND LAWRENCE NUTTALL

Introduction

The scenario presented is an emotive one that raises a number of ethical issues for which there are no easy answers. This commentary will offer reflections in relation to three aspects of the case: 1) the decision not to inform the young man of the fact that he had been taken off the transplant list; 2) the medical decision to remove the young man from the list; and 3) the social worker's dilemma.

Withholding information

The first striking aspect of this case scenario for most social workers will be the fact that the team did not share full and important information with a 19-year-old competent adult. Both medical and social work ethics promote the value of individual autonomy, and certainly social workers believe that the expertise that service users have in regard to their own problems should never be ignored or dismissed; rather, service users should take a significant part in any decision-making process that concerns them. Medical case law in Britain has advanced to a point where patients' rights, especially their rights to make their own choices about issues relevant to their lives (autonomy), are stressed. Autonomy is clearly considered the 'trumping' value (it has the highest ranking) in medical ethics. How could this team justify keeping vital information from a competent young man whose life and death were at stake? Regardless of the concerns expressed by the medical team, it seems that the right of this patient to be a full and active participant in his own care was violated. He was treated paternalistically, and he and his family were disempowered and deprived of crucial information concerning his medical care.

Clearly in this case the medical team prioritised other values over patient autonomy – namely what they saw as the welfare of the young man and of the staff and other patients in the hospital. The medical team in question decided that it was in the 'best interests' of the patient to not inform him of his status. The majority of the team believed that sharing information could lead to a loss of hope for this man, possible depression, and would not in any way contribute to his well-being. Team members also questioned the benefit to the hospital staff and other patients if this young man were to be told he was off the transplant list. Not only was this approach paternalistic (hospital staff thought they knew what was best for the young man), but, by introducing and giving significant weight to the best interests of other patients and the hospital staff, there was a risk that the needs of the patient would be subordinated to those of the institution.

Removal from the waiting list

The preceding discussion is in no way meant to imply that the actual decision to remove the young man from the waiting list was in any way an unfair decision. Certainly, in a climate of limited resources, it is simply a fact that not every patient waiting for an organ will actually be offered one; the medical team does have to make a judgement as to how the available organs are allocated. In this case scenario the decision appears to be consistent with the principles of clinical need and the likelihood of benefit. There is certainly an argument to be made that offering this young man an organ could be considered 'medically futile', since it is broadly agreed that an organ would only increase his lifespan for a few months. From a utilitarian perspective, if we take fairness to be about the distribution of goods to promote the greatest good of the greatest number of people, then this decision was probably a fair one.

The social worker's dilemma

Clearly the social worker is in a difficult position, given that it is necessary to maintain effective working relationships with other professionals in order to advocate on behalf of patients. Nevertheless, the most fundamental duty that the social worker has is toward the patient. Entering into an agreement, albeit reluctantly, with the medical staff not to share crucial information with the patient can be regarded as a dereliction of duty. Should this decision subsequently become known, it would call into question the basis for trust between the social worker and this and other patients. The social worker could potentially be deemed to have brought the profession into disrepute.

The decision by the medical team to withhold vital information from the patient not only has the effect of denying him and his family their due process rights to challenge the decision, it also prevents future patients from benefiting from any successful outcome following on from a challenge. The decision also risks undermining any basis of trust between patients and hospital staff.

Concluding comments

In the final analysis, there does not appear to be a strong argument that the decision to remove the 19-year-old young man from the transplant waiting list was in itself unfair. However, the fundamentally flawed decision not to inform, which denies him the most basic of rights, creates considerable unfairness in that he is being treated differently from the way patients would expect to be treated and this would appear not to be justified. Although the social worker is placed in a very difficult position and is outnumbered by medical staff, in our view there were good ethical arguments that she could draw upon to challenge the medical team in this case and work towards changing attitudes and practices in future similar cases.

Tamara Catchpole Horsburgh, MSW and Juris Doctorate from the University of Maryland. She is pursuing a Ph.D. at Glasgow University, and is a lecturer at the University of the West of Scotland.

Lawrence Nuttall, BA (Hons) Social Work from Reading University and MA Social Policy and Criminology from the Open University, UK. He is studying for a Ph.D. at Stirling University and is a lecturer at the University of the West of Scotland.

Commentary 2

AMY M. CHOW

Medical settings are arenas for lots of difficult decisions based on ethical considerations. With the constant insufficiency of resources for growing demands, decisions about setting limits have to be made. Coupled with the nature of issues related to life and death, the urgency in decision-making, as well as the diversified value orientation of different professionals, a fair decision about resource allocation in a health-care setting usually entails numerous immense struggles within the individual and the team.

The case about the young man waiting for a transplant, which is common in many parts of the world, illustrates these struggles within the social worker and other team members. The struggles were lessened by the existence of a national protocol which offers a clear rationale and evidence in the list of criteria to be considered in the decision-making process. The protocol helps to improve fairness as the criteria are evidence based and consistent across the country. Moreover, it is easily accessible for all from the website, and is subjected to review every two years. The criteria are of wide dimensions and the final decision of placing a patient on the waiting list is based on discussions in a multidisciplinary meeting. The inclusion of views from different professionals also helps to strike a balance of value orientations.

In this case, the controversy seems to be not in the decision of placing or not placing the young man on the waiting list. Though the decision is tough, everyone shows consent that the patient's name has to be removed from the waiting list. The non-eventful decision-making process in this aspect can be attributed to the good foundation set by the national protocol which carries a strong emphasis on fairness.

However, the principle of fairness is not limited to the admission to the waiting list. It should be applied to access to information as well as to participation in the decision-making process. Though the criteria stated in the protocol are accessible on the worldwide web, is the patient aware of the protocol? Would there be a chance that other ethnic groups who have limited understanding of English would not be able to comprehend the content? For special groups who have barriers in using computers, can they access this piece of information through other means? If not, the fairness principle is not completely applied. Access to this piece of information can help prepare the patients to work on criteria that can be modifiable – for example, body mass index, compliance with medical treatment or smoking. Withholding this piece of information might take away the young man's chance of being placed on the waiting list. In addition, the information that names can be taken off the waiting list according to medical condition is also withheld from the patient. Probably the withholding of information might reduce some immediate problems, but it might cause complications in future. Fairness in participation is my concern too. I wonder whether the process of discussion should include the patient, or at least offer him a chance to choose to join in a discussion or not? The decision-making process is led by a group of health care professionals. Are we assuming professional knowledge guarantees the best knowledge about this patient? Should his view be considered?

The major controversy about this case concerns the breaking of bad news. This controversy will be removed if the young man is a participant in the multidisciplinary meeting. Yet, going back to the situation in this case, the social worker is facing great challenges in upholding her belief in patients' rights to know about their condition. This is again related to the principle of fairness. Is it fair for professionals to take away patients' rights to plan for the use of their days towards the end of their lives? Are we really in a better position to understand their needs? The death by suicide of another patient after receiving bad news is alarming, but is it fair to generalise to all other patients as well?

The social worker in this case has respected the team decision and tried her best to share her views as a team member. This is an optimal way to work on the case. Coming from Hong Kong with a Chinese background, I think the case might be further complicated in our context. Our protocol is not openly available to the public as it is in the United Kingdom. In addition, a decision made by family members is sometimes of higher importance than that of the patient. However, a consensus among all family members is not often found in reality. The family dynamics can put extra pressure on the process of care. Moreover, we are facing an extra challenge in handling cases of organ transplant in Hong Kong. There seem to be illegal supplies of organs from nearby countries, which can be purchased. Some patients might take this chance, if they can afford the cost. Is it fair that those who have money have a higher chance of getting an organ transplant? Is it fair for the organ donors in other countries, which usually have lower living standards?

There are no easy answers to the questions, but discussion among team members, and even among society, can help us in approaching the issue. The setting up of the protocol in the UK is a good example of how evidence-based and open protocols can help to reduce some unnecessary dilemmas among team members. Regular clinical supervision is also helpful for social workers who have personal dilemmas. Inspired by this case, I think we can extend our multiple roles as social workers. Taking on the role of advocates we can extend our work in fighting for the rights of service users and patients to information and participation in the decision-making process. As social work educators, we can promote psycho-educational programmes about organ donation, to reduce the competition for donated organs.

Amy M. Chow is a Chinese Assistant Professor at the University of Hong Kong. Her first job was as a medical social worker in a general hospital. She has worked as a bereavement counsellor in a community-based counselling centre, and has extensive work experience in hospice settings as well.

Questions for discussion about Case 4.2

1 What do you think is the key ethical issue in this case and how is it related to fairness?
2 The second commentator raises two important questions: a) Is it fair for professionals to take away patients' rights to plan for the use of their days towards the end of their lives?; and b) Are we (professionals) really in a better position to understand their needs? Discuss these questions, if possible bringing in your own professional experience.
3 Rules and norms about organ transplants are not the same all over the world. What is the situation in your country? Can you think of ethical guidelines for this complicated issue that would help fair decision-making?

Case 4.3 Dilemmas in working with a gypsy family: a story from a Portuguese social educator

Introduction

This case is about a dilemma faced by a male social educator ('educador social') working with a gypsy community ('etnia cigana') in a large Portuguese city. In Portugal, social educators are qualified professional practitioners who combine a social and pedagogical approach to social problems and community-based intervention. In this sense, their role has some similarities with community and youth workers in Britain, and social pedagogues and special educators in other parts of Europe. They are able to work with different social groups such as children, young people, adults and older people. In Portugal, the term 'etnia cigana' is used to refer to nomad communities with origins in different European countries with specific cultural and social backgrounds. We have used the English translation 'gypsy community', as opposed to the more politically correct term 'travelling community', as this captures both the nomadic and cultural aspects of 'etnia cigana'.

The case

Miguel is an experienced social educator who works for the Commission for the Protection of Children and Young People (*Comissão de Protecção de Crianças e Jovens*) in a large Portuguese city. He has been assigned to work with the social team and teachers in a public secondary school. In Portugal, children must stay in school until they are 16 years old and children's families must be able to ensure them this fundamental right. If children start failing or quitting school, the Commission is brought in to start an intervention with children's families, working alongside them to ensure the necessary conditions (such as access to health care) are in place for the families in order for the children to stay in school.

The school where Miguel is working is located in a deprived urban area characterised by strong dynamics of social exclusion and poverty. This is an area with high rates of unemployment; low levels of educational qualifications; the greatest concentration of social housing projects in the city; a significant population of ethnic minorities, with social integration issues; high rates of youth crime and teenage pregnancy; low access to cultural and social infrastructures within communities; high school drop-out rates before the end of compulsory school; and criminality related to drugs trafficking.

Miguel is based in a team developing projects to ensure children and young people stay in school and succeed in their studies, alongside intervention with their families in the community. The presence of a significant number of children and young people from gypsy communities led the school to develop a specific intervention with them. This comprises special learning support for individual pupils from teachers and the social work team; special curriculum adaptation that would enable students to learn different subjects; and social and cultural projects to address the gypsy culture and history within the school in order to address social discrimination issues.

Miguel has developed an educational project in the community to reduce school drop outs. In order to do this he needed to integrate himself in the community and has developed an intensive programme of work explaining the importance of school and education in a citizen's life.

One of the families Miguel is working with is the Silva family. This family comprises two parents who work as merchants at fairs and three children: a girl called Gloria (15 years old) and two boys aged 11 and 9 years old. He has been working with this family for five years.

Gloria was promised, at birth, to marry a gypsy man by her father. Gloria had a brilliant school record. According to her culture, at the age of puberty she would have to drop out of school so she would not be in contact with other men and had the possibility of keeping herself 'pure' for her future husband. Gloria reached puberty at the age of 13. However, as a result of Miguel's work, the gypsy community leader authorised Gloria to remain at school after the age of 13. This was due to the fact that the community leader respected Miguel for all the good work he had done in the community.

However, today, Gloria is 15 years old and is getting married. Her future husband belongs to a different community and will probably not authorise her to carry on with school, even though it is Gloria's wish. She asked desperately for Miguel's help to talk to the community leader. Miguel is hesitant and unsure how to proceed. On the one hand he wants to meet Gloria's needs and her desire to stay in school, since he knows how important it is for her. On the other hand, he is concerned that if he does raise this with the leader it might be seen as a lack of respect to the gypsy culture. Miguel is afraid of losing all the trust built during years of permanence in the community. Miguel recognises the need to respect cultural features of the community, namely, the role of women and the social rule of marriage at that age. Even though Miguel has a good relationship with the community leader, he does not want to show disrespect towards his culture.

Commentary 1

ADALBERTO DIAS DE CARVALHO, ANA MARIA SERAPICOS, FLORBELA SAMAGAIO, GABRIELA TREVISAN, WALTER ALMEIDA, ÁLVARO FARIA AND IGOR MAGALHÃES

Social and policy background

Before discussing the ethical issues involved in this case, it is important to outline some features of the social, cultural and policy context in which it is located. The presented case took place in a deprived area of a Portuguese city. In Portugal, the Ministry of Education has designated most of these areas as Educational Territories of Primary Intervention (*Territórios Educativos de Intervenção Priotitária*). In these areas, social intervention is conceived holistically – joining schools, health services, childcare protection and family services, cultural institutions, community centres, employment centres, adult learning and training centres and other community resources in order to address the different problems in each community.

The specific focus of this case is a gypsy family. Gypsy communities have a rich and ancient culture, with very specific social roles for everyone inside the communities. Men are responsible for taking care of family and other community members, particularly the elderly who have a very important role. Community leaders are usually older people, who are considered wiser. Community decisions are frequently discussed with them and decisions made based upon their opinions. As for children, they attend school, especially when it comes to primary school, where they learn how to read and write. Boys usually stay in school for a longer time than girls. For children, marriage is usually decided before they are born, when they are promised to marry another gypsy boy or girl. When girls become 'women', that is when they first menstruate, that means that they should be kept in the community in order to keep themselves pure for marriage. Culturally, it is very important to keep marriages inside gypsy communities and families. When they leave school, youngsters usually start helping their parents in fairs, learning their job and becoming increasingly considered as adults, especially after getting married. Nevertheless, it is important not to stereotype gypsy culture. We can find many different types of gypsy communities, some of which are quite open to the possibility of studying and even to the idea of university education for both men and woman. Even so, most remain conscious of their cultural history and background, and are keen to preserve it.

Regarding official projects, Portugal has a High Commission for Immigration and Intercultural Dialogue (ACIDI) that addresses specifically the gypsy communities, supporting different integration and non-discrimination projects. At the present time, gypsy communities face a lot of different kinds of discrimination, mainly based on cultural differences from the mainstream Portuguese and on the ways of living (mainly characterised as merchants at fairs, for instance).

The ethical issues

The case ends with the presentation of the dilemma facing Miguel. We do not know how he resolves this, but we could disentangle some of the ethical issues and arguments involved.

The main ethical challenge present in this case lies in Miguel's effort to keep his relationship with the community and, at the same time, to attend to Gloria's own needs and expectations. For Miguel, the building of this relationship with the community was hard work and he managed to achieve different goals while working with them. If Miguel breaks this relationship, it will be hard to recapture; at the same time, he needs to address Gloria's expectations regarding school and her own future. The two cultures have different, but equally valid, perspectives on school and on teenagers' lives. Miguel is able to understand them. His focus, however, is on Gloria's well-being and future, and that implies that she can 'break' with some strong cultural aspects of her community.

On Miguel's side, the main concern is, then, to be able to respect both sides and find a solution that would satisfy them. He still needs to work alongside the community leader and have his permission so that Gloria can stay in school. For the community leader, issues of protection and culture arise if Gloria stays in school. For Gloria, staying in school means having the chance to learn more and have a different future than the one prescribed for her by her community. Could Miguel try to revisit the leader's position regarding Gloria's school continuance, assuring him that she would still comply with her own culture and, at the same time, be able to stay at school? Could he try engaging in a new relationship with Gloria's future husband and seek his approval?

On the other hand, a key argument when discussing intervention with minority communities has to do with balancing children's fundamental rights, especially when they conflict with each other, such as the right to education versus the right to culture and personal heritage. The choice – if there is one to be made at all – has delicate features that could compromise the social educator's position, not only within the community but also with Gloria, who has expectations and aspirations about attending school.

The two positions (the right to education versus the right to culture) seem, at a first glance, incompatible. However, there are ways of dealing with gypsy children's cultural backgrounds and the need to keep them at school for the longest possible period of time. Some public schools in Portugal have created special classes exclusively for children from gypsy communities. The main argument is that this is a way of both respecting the concerns of the community and, at the same time, including children in school. This solution avoids undesirable mixing between non-gypsy boys and/or girls. This solution, however, is not satisfactory for everyone. From a basic ethical standpoint it could be argued that this increases the segregation of the gypsy community. From another perspective, however, it could be argued that it is best to have them in school, where they can stay for a longer period of time and develop their learning skills and knowledge. A third perspective could be to consider the possibility of keeping children in the community, but also maintaining school learning, if the school could come to the community and teach the children and young people.

Whatever approach is taken, Miguel's position is not easy and there are no quick fixes. For he has to consider many perspectives: the gypsy community; the child protection services; the need to respect individual rights (Gloria's rights to schooling but also to her cultural and social heritage); and the need to respect collective rights (both of schools and communities).

Adalberto Dias de Carvalho is Professor at ESEPF and ISCET, a researcher at the University of Porto and Head of the Social Education Department of ESEPF, Portugal.
Ana Maria Serapicos is Professor at ESEPF and practicum supervisor.
Florbela Samagaio is Professor at ESEPF and practicum supervisor.
Gabriela Trevisan is Professor at ESEPF, assistant to the Head of the Social Education Department of ESEPF and practicum supervisor.
Walter Almeida is Professor at ESEPF and practicum supervisor.
Álvaro Faria is a social educator at SOS children's villages project.
Igor Magalhães is a social educator, Instituto Profissional do Terço.

Commentary 2

VIVIENNE BOZALEK

The key ethical issues in this case

The ethical issues in this case concern the dilemma of the social pedagogical worker, Miguel, about whether or not to approach the community
leader on behalf of Gloria, who is 15 years old and is having to drop out
of school because she is getting married to a gypsy man to whom she
was promised at birth. Gloria, who has a 'brilliant school record', has
asked Miguel to intervene with the community leader on her behalf, as
it is her wish to stay at school. Miguel's dilemma is that he is not sure
how to proceed – he is aware of the importance of staying at school for
Gloria and her need and desire in this regard, but he is also aware of the
cultural imperatives of the role of women in the community and their
social rules of marriage. He does not want to disrespect the cultural values
of the community nor interfere with the good relationship that he has
built up with the community leader.

Miguel works for the Commission for the Protection of Children and
Young People so his first priority should be the best interests of this
particular group of people in the community in which he works. It is a
fundamental right for children in Portugal to stay at school until they are
16 years of age, and the Commission is called in to work with families
to ensure that children do not leave before this age. There is a very clear
path for Miguel with regard to this case – both the national right to
education until the age of 16 years and the mandate of the Commission
to intervene with families regarding this matter to ensure that children
remain at school until this age. Miguel should therefore place the needs
of Gloria above those of the culture of the community, as he is in the
community specifically to advocate for the rights of children to remain
in school until they are 16 years old.

Examining the fairness of this case from social justice perspectives

This case could be viewed from two different approaches which examine
the fairness of situations – i.e., from social justice perspectives. Two
perspectives that offer fruitful potential for considering the fairness of
this particular case are the human capabilities perspective as developed

by Amartya Sen (1992, 1999, 2009) and Martha Nussbaum (2000, 2006); and Nancy Fraser's (2009) approach to social justice, which offers a gendered perspective.

The human capabilities approach looks at what people are actually able to do, and able to be, and how they are able to choose the different types of lives they have reason to value as contributing to their well-being (Sen 2009). In our example, Gloria values being educated. The human capabilities approach would regard it as important for Gloria to have the choice to pursue this goal of education as contributing to her well-being as a person. As Alkire and Deneulin (2009: 40) state: 'In order to be agents of their own lives, people need the freedom to be educated, to speak in public without fear, to have freedom of expression and association, etc.'

From a human capabilities perspective, being fair would also mean regarding each person as an end in themselves rather than a means to an end – that each person should be regarded as equally worthy as the next person (Nussbaum 2000). The human capabilities approach focuses on the opportunities that are available (i.e., what people are able to do and to be) to flourish as human beings. The goal of social justice from this perspective is human flourishing for each and every person. This means that Gloria should be regarded as a person in her own right rather than as a means to an end. Sacrificing her education for marriage to appease the cultural expectations of her community would be regarded as unfair. Gloria's ability to flourish as a human being would be compromised should she have to give up her educational career for that of marriage. Nussbaum (2006: 322) has noted that 'Education is the key to all human capabilities', and she also alerts us to the fact that women have been regarded too often as caregivers for the family rather than as ends in themselves (Nussbaum 2000).

Regarding Miguel's concern about the culture of the community in which he is working and his desire not to alienate the community leader, Nussbaum would regard this as unfair or unjust. He would be seen to be deferring to currently powerful men in the community, rather than listening to the voices of women or the voices of dissent and contestation regarding women's and children's rights to education.

From a feminist or gendered perspective, this situation would certainly not be regarded as a fair one – it would be considered as an instance of gendered injustice. Fraser (2009) outlines three distinct dimensions of gender injustice or unfairness: cultural, economic and political. For Gloria to relinquish her education to appease the imperatives in her community for the marriage that has been arranged for her would be regarded as unjust in the cultural dimension, and perhaps in a more indirect way, in both the economic and political dimensions as well. This is because education has a direct bearing on the sorts of employment Gloria would be able to secure in the future, expanding her options for social agency, and would impact on her ability to represent herself politically and have her voice heard. Fraser comments that there is no good in transforming culture without transforming social institutions.

Concluding comments

Both the human capabilities approach and Fraser's tri-valent notion of social justice foreground the importance of considering social arrangements in being able to achieve human flourishing, well-being and participatory parity. It would thus be important for a social pedagogue such as Miguel to ensure that social arrangements and conditions exist to protect the right of girls and young women to receive education. This would be important for their well-being and their ability to participate as full human beings on an equal footing with others.

References

Alkire, S. and Deneulin, S. (2009) 'The human capability and development approach', in S. Deneulin and L. Shahan (eds) *An Introduction to the Human Development and Capability Approach: Freedom and Agency*, London: Earthscan.

Fraser, N. (2009) 'Feminism, capitalism and the cunning of history', *New Left Review*, 56: 97–117.

Nussbaum, M. (2000) *Women and Human Development*, Cambridge, MA: Cambridge University Press.

Nussbaum, M. (2006) 'Education and democratic citizenship: capabilities and equality education', *Journal of Human Development*, 7(3): 385–398.

Sen, A. (1992) *Inequality Re-examined*, Oxford: Oxford University Press.

Sen, A. (1999) *Development as Freedom*, New York: Alfred Knopf.

Sen, A. (2009) *The Idea of Justice*, Cambridge, MA: The Belknap Press of Harvard University Press.

Vivienne Bozalek is a Professor of Social Work and holds a Ph.D. from Utrecht University. Her Ph.D. looked at issues of social justice and the political ethics of care. She was Chairperson of the Social Work Department of the University of the Western Cape (UWC) in Cape Town, South Africa, but has been seconded into the position of Director of Teaching and Learning at UWC, an historically disadvantaged university.

Questions for discussion about Case 4.3

1 Where do you think the 'unfairness' lies in this case? Do you think separate provision of services (including schooling and social services) for ethnic and cultural minority groups is a good way of promoting fairness in society?

2 How much weight do you think should be given to respecting a community's 'culture' in cases like this? Can you relate this case to similar cases in your own experience of working with minority groups?

3 How would you characterise Miguel's role in this case – as an advocate (for Gloria or for the gypsy community) and/or as a mediator (between Gloria and the community leader or the gypsy community and wider society) or in some other way? What do you think his role should be?

Case study 4.4

Case 4.4   A gay applicant who wants to adopt a child: a case from Turkey

Introduction

This case was written by a social worker who works for the Social Services Directorate in a Turkish city. In Turkey, the Social Services Directorate is a governmental body which delivers, coordinates, regulates and controls all the social services. This is a central institution with branches in all the cities and some districts. The case concerns the request by a gay man to adopt a child. In Turkey, the general attitude towards being gay is that it is either an illness or a deviation. Despite declarations in the 1970s that homosexuality is not a pathology and should not be taken as a criterion for discrimination, public tolerance for the acceptance of homosexuality in Turkish society is generally low. Lesbian, gay, bisexual and transgender people (LGBT) still face various types of pressure, including discrimination, abuse, assault and hate crimes. In Turkey, the family is accepted as the basic social unit, typically conceived of in terms of heterosexual relationships.

The case

Ahmet was a 32-year-old university graduate who was gay. He worked in the private sector as a computer programmer. He wanted to use the adoption service to adopt a boy. His socio-economic conditions were good enough to allow for the healthy development and care of a child.

Ahmet applied to the Social Services Directorate in the city where he lived. His application was dealt with by a female social worker who had been working for three years especially in the fields of adoption and child protection. After detailed social assessments and interviews, it was decided by the social worker that his circumstances were sufficient to fulfil the criteria for being an adoptive parent. Turkish marital law says: 'If an unmarried person is over 30 years of age, he or she can adopt on his or her own.' Previously the age limit had been 35 years, but the law was changed and the age limit was dropped to 30 years, and single people were also able to adopt. These points were all in Ahmet's favour. In the law the term 'person' is used. There are no clear references to a person's sexual orientation, which was also an important factor in Ahmet's case.

In this situation, however, the social worker faced a dilemma. Should she decide that Ahmet could access the adoption service, since he was clearly eligible according to the criteria expressed in the law? Alternatively, should she decide that a child should not live with a gay parent, since he might endanger 'the best interests of the child' – which should be the social worker's primary concern according to the United Nations Convention on the Rights of the Child? If the social worker acted according to the ethical principles of unconditional acceptance of the applicant as an individual, who should not be mistreated or discriminated against, then she should allow the adoption to take place. However, the social worker felt that the nurturing of the potential adopted child in a 'healthy' family environment would be risked in the event of deciding that the applicant could adopt. The social worker judged that the school, friends and social environment of the child would be in chaos, and this would be traumatic for the child. Another issue that the social worker worried about was the fact that there would be a risk that the child might be confused about the development of his own sexual identity. There would be a probability of the child taking his parent as a model in terms of his sexual development. The general views and feedback from the social workers' colleagues in the agency setting informally suggested that she should not allow the applicant to adopt; this would not be in accordance with the best interests of the child.

The social worker went through the ethical dilemma described here and could not decide whether she should let the applicant adopt or not.

She thought about both options, and the positive and negative results they would produce. She decided not to let Ahmet adopt a child. This was not a decision that the social worker liked very much. However, she felt she knew and understood very well the country's culture and prevailing social attitudes. She thought that she acted in the best interests of the potential adopted child.

The social worker tried to explain the reasons behind the refusal to Ahmet. She told him that the dominant social and cultural patterns and the general attitudes and stereotypes in society against homosexuality would not grant him the right to adoption. In addition, the social worker tried to explain her worry that the child's sexual development in a 'healthy' climate might be threatened and her concern about possible problems he would be exposed to in the home environment. Ahmet had to control his anger and disappointment, and was well-prepared and calm enough to hear the negative answer, since he himself had suffered the discrimination the social worker had referred to as a reason for turning down his application. Nevertheless, this was a total disappointment for him. He knew that he could insist and go to the court to assert his rights – since it was not the law but the social worker's own worries that had resulted in the rejection of his application. However, he did not feel he could pursue the case any further since he was well aware of the social pressures. Most likely, he had every right to adopt a child; and following the rejection of his application he knew that he could go on and battle to overturn the decision in court. But the problem was not only about laws and regulations in a country, it was also about the deep seeds of discrimination against those regarded as 'other'.

Commentary 1

AGNES VERBRUGGEN

The process of writing a commentary on this case has been quite challenging for me. I found that the case got under my skin and troubled me, so I discussed it with several people. From this process of discussion, thinking and writing I feel I learnt something important about how to handle ethical problems and dilemmas.

- To be able and willing to engage in dialogue with others about ethical problems helps us to make better decisions. To deliberate about our ethical standards as applied to a real case brings in the complexity, the shades of grey between the black and white assumptions.

- We can 'solve' ethical problems as 'experts' – so called 'autonomous' thinkers. However, solving an ethical problem is something different from *experiencing* an ethical dilemma. In order to experience an ethical dilemma, it is necessary to get involved in a case. Getting involved is about searching for that action that fits the vision of the person/social worker that I want to be.

I see three possible decisions that the social worker could make in this case, which I will now evaluate.

1 No adoption allowed

The interests of the child are of greater importance than the wish of Ahmet to raise a child. The rationale for this choice is based on taking into account the consequences of the adoption. Since Ahmet belongs to a minority group that experiences discrimination in his culture, he is not the 'right' person to give a child full chances for a healthy development. Another possible reason for not allowing the adoption is that raising a child is a long-term engagement and therefore it might be careless to leave this to just one person. The 'privatisation' of the relationship between parents and their children (that is, seeing the main rights and responsibilities in relation to child care as a private family matter rather than a matter of public concern) leads to children becoming regarded as personal projects – as meaning-makers for adults. Therefore it becomes very important for people to have children 'of their own'. Parents seem to have the exclusive moral and pedagogical authority over 'their' children. This is too narrow a basis for parenthood and prevents a broader natural foundation for raising children. There is an African proverb: 'In order to raise a child, you need a whole village.'

This solution for the case leaves some questions.

The first question is: Who decides the criteria for judging what are 'good' consequences – Ahmet or the social worker? Secondly, since human behaviour is (fortunately) never completely predictable, how can we foresee all the consequences? Another problem is that the argument used to discriminate against Ahmet in not allowing the adoption is based on the fact that he belongs to a minority group that is discriminated against. This is not only a circular argument, it is also neither fair, nor socially just. However, it is a reality in Turkey that gay, lesbian and bisexual people face discrimination. There is a cultural gap between the law (the state) and the mores of 'civil society'. However, justice as fairness requires compensation for the inequalities between people due to historical and social circumstances. Certainly social workers – as representatives of the state – have to take a stand against these inequalities.

Conclusion: a simple 'no' to Ahmet's application is unfair and socially unjust.

2 Allow adoption

The social worker cannot deny or overrule the marital law. Ahmet fits all the criteria and the social investigation of his circumstances (what he can provide for the child) should have a positive outcome. The justification for this decision is based on rationally grounded and democratic principles: autonomy and equity; that is, everyone, without discrimination, should have access to the same 'sources of happiness'.

This action also leaves unanswered questions.

Allowing adoption because Ahmet fulfils all the 'objective' criteria may not take into account what reasons or motives Ahmet has for adopting a child. This approach to decision-making can be very careless, even unsafe, for the adopted child. Human rights are perceived as a protection against externally imposed forces, but they are not a protection against moral critique. The fact that someone has rights does not mean that they can exercise these rights without any limits. If we seek to answer the question about what the limits should be within a legal framework, the result is the following polarisation. People should be left alone to do what they want; the only 'good' reason to interfere is when they are harming, or likely to harm, others. On this basis, the only reason to interfere would be on the grounds of safety, not care. This is a particular problem for social workers, since their work is about taking care that the right thing is done for everyone involved. Their role is about taking care of fairness.

Conclusion: simply allowing adoption is unfair and socially unjust.

3 Allow adoption if certain conditions are fulfilled

A third option is that the social worker starts with confirmation that the adoption is legally permissible, but delays making a definitive decision.

First, some questions must be explored in dialogue with Ahmet. The rationale for this option is a dialogue-based approach to ethics. It would involve considering the question: What does 'allowing' adoption really mean? Arguably the answer is that it means that through the social worker the state assigns a parent-child relationship between Ahmet and the child. This *is* distributive justice. It is the government that gives social recognition to the specific relation between this adult and this child. This means that social justice is about more than maximising the greatest happiness for the greatest number of people (option 1); and about more than giving people freedom of choice (option 2). This means that equity between people is always a hypothetical assumption, which has to be realised in a concrete, real situation.

Therefore, the answer to the question, 'What is socially just?', *cannot* be found only by (finding principles for) distributing goods in a just way. Social justice is about *the right way to value and measure social goods*. In order to value social goods we must know their purpose. What is the purpose of the institutionalisation of the relationship between (adoptive) parents and (adopted) children? There is never an *a priori* answer to that question, because it evolves as a result of a societal process and the answer must be given within the particular context of a real situation.

Therefore, in making a moral judgement about this case, the social worker has to make an assessment, taking into account Ahmet's concrete situation, of the value for Ahmet and for the child of approving the officially recognised adoptive parenthood. Within a confidential relationship, Ahmet and the social worker must deliberate about doing the right thing for everyone involved: Ahmet, the child and the broader society.

Conclusion: this dialogical process seems the best guarantee for a fair and just decision.

Agnes Verbruggen is a social worker, sociologist and Master in Law. She teaches professional ethics to social workers and supervises students at Hogeschool Gent, Belgium. Her teaching is inspired by the concept of the sociological imagination and by Socrates, Habermas and Nussbaum.

Commentary 2

ANA M. SOBOČAN

Ethical issues and value conflicts are pervasive in the field of child welfare. Social workers are confronted with cases that are often fraught with uncertainties. Accurate predictions of the child protection risks present big challenges and generate dilemmas against a background of conflicting obligations and directives. Social workers have to strive towards determining the best interests of the child, while at the same time refraining from imposing cultural values and beliefs on families and individuals from diverse backgrounds.

The assumed best interests of the child seem also to be at the core of this case. A social worker has found herself in a dilemma between protecting what she believes is beneficial and non-harmful for a child and the legal right of a person, who meets the eligibility criteria, to adopt a child. At the core of her decision lies the anticipated attitude towards the potential adopted child, who would be living with a homosexual parent. Her main concerns are attitudes in society and the sexual development of the child.

The debate about whether to place children with homosexual adoptive parents is ongoing, and will continue to exist as long as there are conflicting views about homosexuality. Social workers and other professionals working in the adoption field need to be aware of their own personal prejudices and beliefs that inform their judgements. Western research has shown that there are no significant differences between children who grow up with heterosexual parents and those raised by homosexual parents – not in their sexual orientation, social adjustment or any other characteristic. Similarly, research has demonstrated that the gender of parents does not influence the well-being of a child. There is a widespread professional consensus on the positive outcomes for children growing up with homosexual parents.

Despite the fact that research undertaken in the Western world clearly supports adoption by homosexual people, in this particular case there are more issues to be considered. We may begin by considering the Turkish legal system, which obviously does not prohibit adoption by homosexual or single people. This view is supported also in the context of the professional stance of social work in Turkey. The document *Ethical Principles and Responsibilities of Social Workers* (published by the Association of Social Workers in Turkey) explicitly directs social workers to provide the best possible service to clients, regardless of (among other factors) sexual orientation or social status, and prohibits them from practising or facilitating any form of discrimination on the basis of (among other factors) sexual orientation or marital status. Social workers are instructed to support an environment in which respect for cultural and social differences is generated.

On the other hand, what hinders the social worker in this case in making a positive decision regarding Ahmet is her view of the sociocultural context and the anticipated attitude towards this issue in the organisation where she is employed. Her decision must be considered in the framework of the social context, the moral guidance stemming from the social identity/ position she holds herself, the responses of her colleagues and the environment in which she is practising. I believe it is possible that in some countries an unfavourable decision in the case of a homosexual adoption applicant would initiate accusations of homophobia and discrimination. Similarly, a positive decision in this case by the Turkish social worker might place her in a position where she would be unfavourably judged and find herself unsupported by her colleagues and community. In my view, taking too much account of the views of colleagues and the wider community in the decision-making process is not in accordance with the role of a professional social worker, no matter how understandable it is.

According to the information given here, and based on similar experiences in other countries, we can to a large extent anticipate what the final outcome of the application process will be. For whatever decision an individual social worker might make to approve a homosexual man as a potential adoptive parent, there are systems in operation which mean, in reality, that such adoptions are not supported structurally. Therefore, there is little chance of someone like Ahmet, who has been approved as an adoptive parent, actually having the possibility of adopting a child. Nevertheless, one of the widely accepted and confirmed findings of the literature on justice is that people can accept negative, unfavourable or disappointing outcomes if they have experienced a fair process in which these outcomes were arrived at by an objective, egalitarian and non-discriminatory approach.

From this perspective, my view on this particular case is that the social worker's conduct and decision should be focused on the actual assessment of whether the applicant is capable of becoming a parent to a child in need of parents. Has the social worker sought the applicant's own views on the implications of homosexual identity and parental identity in the Turkish context? Has she explored his future plans and resilience strategies regarding homosexual parenting? Has she investigated his resources and social networks which would support his parental role? If Ahmet is able to meet the needs of an individual child and to develop a child's strengths, in my opinion the social worker should proceed with approving Ahmet as a suitable adoptive parent. However, at the same time she should explain and clearly state to the applicant what are the actual and realistic possibilities of a positive final outcome (that is, how likely it is that he will succeed in adopting a child).

Reference

Association of Social Workers in Turkey (no date) *Ethical Principles and Responsibilities of Social Workers* (English version), Ankara: ASWT, available at http://www.ifsw.org/p38000300.html

Ana M. Sobočan, M.A, is a researcher and assistant lecturer in the Faculty of Social Work at the University of Ljubljana, Slovenia. She has conducted research on topics such as foster care, (international) adoptions and social parenthood, as well as same-sex families in Slovenia.

Questions for discussion about Case 4.4

1 What do you think are the main ethical issues in this case?
2 Do you think it was fair to Ahmet and/or to the male children waiting for adoption that the social worker refused Ahmet's application to be an adoptive parent?
3 What kinds of ethical arguments would be most persuasive for you in judging whether the social worker's decision was right or wrong?

Challenging and developing organisations

Introduction

DONNA McAULIFFE

This chapter presents a number of cases that illustrate the complexities of the organisational context of practice. Social welfare and human services operate as a multifaceted 'industry' in most countries, governed by a plethora of laws, policies and jurisdictions, as well as cultural and social mores, that dictate how people should relate to each other, and what duties, responsibilities and obligations should be observed. In the professional context, it is expected that practitioners who have public accountability will abide by both the ethics of the profession and the standards of conduct mandated by the employing organisational authority. These standards may or may not have a basis in law, and there are distinct differences internationally about the regulation of behaviour and what can be done about practitioners who breach established codes of ethics. The cases in this chapter illustrate what can happen when social workers and others in helping professions have responsibility for the interpretation of organisational policies that may stand in opposition to a legislative requirement (Case 5.2 about social care insurance in Peru), and the implications of role conflict or differences in value positions when people working together do not share common understandings of ethical practice (Cases 5.1, 5.3 and 5.4). The questions that these cases raise include:

- What is the organisational context in which social work practice operates, and what challenges does this present in terms of ethos and culture?
- How far should social workers go in advocating for policy change on social justice grounds within an organisational context that might be hostile to valid critique?
- How do people work together in multi-professional and inter-professional contexts, when there are value conflicts or differing interpretations of ethical standards, policies or laws?
- What are the responsibilities and obligations that social workers have to colleagues, and how is unethical conduct challenged?

The organisational context of social work

Social work practice generally takes place within the context of some type of organisational structure. There are many ways of describing these human service organisations, and one of these is to divide them up into government or public agencies, 'third sector' organisations (NGOs), and 'private-for-profit' organisations (Chenoweth and McAuliffe 2008: 181). Many social workers are employed in large, bureaucratic, statutory authorities with responsibility for areas such as health, mental health or disability, child and family services, income support, housing or immigration. There are typically many layers of hierarchical management and accountability requirements are high. Social workers are expected to comply with often rigid policies and protocols designed to standardise service delivery in an effort to ensure consistency and equity. Strict requirements for compliance with eligibility assessments, justification of decisions and documentation of practice are commonplace in the interests of public accountability, as these government or public organisations are often funded from taxpayer contributions, and therefore subject to public scrutiny. The organisations featured in Cases 5.1, 5.2 and 5.4 are all in the public sector. The 'third sector' comprises those agencies that are community-based, not-for-profit or self-governing, although they often receive funding from government and are therefore also accountable for public monies. Social workers in third sector agencies may have more autonomy and are more able, because of their external position, to challenge oppressive government policies that might contribute to inequities in the provision of health services, housing and financial support for disadvantaged people. Faith-based organisations also fall into this category (as illustrated by the church-based counselling service in Case 5.3), as do large international aid organisations like World Vision and the Red Cross. Private-for-profit organisations are those that charge fees for services and straddle the human service and business sectors. This would include those social workers who work in their own self-managed private practice environment, or who engage in contract work on behalf of an organisation (although they would still be accountable to an organisational entity by virtue of a contractual agreement).

In thinking about these different types of organisational structures, and in reflecting on the cases presented in this chapter, it can be seen that social workers, as employees or employers, inevitably become part of an organisational culture that may, or may not, have values that are in line with the espoused values of the profession. Where the mission statement of a human services or welfare organisation is clearly about social justice, human rights, responding to needs, alleviating disadvantage, promoting inclusion, respecting diversity and difference, or ensuring that resources are distributed with fairness and equity, social workers will find a more comfortable fit with the ethos and culture. If, however, the organisational mandate is more about economic imperatives, risk identification, managerial structures, productivity and growth at the expense of human need, and distribution of resources based on competition and compliance, social workers may find a more difficult value-fit in their workplace. Practitioners need to be able to reflect on their own personal and professional values and make wise decisions about employment options by using this self-awareness. If a social worker applies for a job in an in-patient mental health unit, but has strong negative attitudes towards use of psychotropic medications, this could result in value clashes with other members of staff. If a social worker who has a religious affiliation that views homosexuality as pathological applies for work in a HIV/AIDS programme (where many of the service users are gay men), this could also be problematic. Social workers need to be able to consider how congruent their own values will be with the values of the organisation for which they work. Case 5.3 is interesting in this respect as it features a social worker who chose to work in a church-based organisation because of his personal faith, but in the end he left because the organisational ethos and practice clashed with his professional values as a social worker.

Brody (2005) has discussed the importance of organisational culture and its influence on the behaviour of staff. There are six factors, he argues, that contribute to organisational stress. These are: role ambiguity; overload (or under-load) of work; contradictory expectations; poor planning; a laid-back atmosphere; and a poor match between staff and jobs. Some of these factors are certainly evident in the cases in this chapter, not just in Case 5.3 about the church-based social worker, but also Cases 5.1 and 5.2 (where contradictory expectations seem to have been placed on staff in a state-run social care institution in Iran and a social insurance agency in Peru).

Working in multi- and inter-professional contexts

Not only do social workers have to consider the organisational culture and what this means for practice, they also have to work alongside many people who have backgrounds in either related or distinctly different professional disciplines. There are various levels of working with other professionals, from multi-professional (collaboration of different professionals) to inter-professional (integration and some interchangeability of professional roles) (Banks with others 2010). The challenges of the multi-professional context and skills required to work effectively in teams where inter-professional working is required cannot be underestimated. Banks (2004: 7) describes inter-professional working as a 'developing trend for members of different professional groups to work together in teams, services, partnerships or taskforces to tackle particularly intractable problems or develop new services'. Reel and Hutchings (2007: 137) have developed the concept of inter-professional working, defining it as:

> a collaborative venture in which those involved share the common purpose of developing mutually negotiated goals which are achieved through agreed care plans and procedures . . . for this to occur, teams need to pool their knowledge and expertise . . . and make joint decisions based upon shared professional view points.

The concept of the multi-professional team is one very common in the health care field, where social workers have taken their place alongside medical and nursing staff and other allied health workers such as psychologists, occupational therapists, speech pathologists, dieticians, pharmacists and physiotherapists. In other contexts, such as international aid organisations, social workers might be working alongside defence personnel, clergy, public health officials, philanthropists, police, journalists, interpreters and cultural advisors. For the most part, the value positions of those dedicated to working in human services will follow the mantra of 'do no harm', with related commitment to ethical principles of autonomy, confidentiality and privacy, professional integrity, respect for persons, and duty of care. Even so, there will always be the potential for differences of opinion between like-minded professionals about what values should take primary importance, particularly when ethical dilemmas are present that challenge personal values. Sound processes of ethical decision-making within an organisational culture of ethical rigour become important so that all professional values and opinions, as well as those that are more personal, can be examined with a view to reaching a mutually agreed position (McAuliffe 2010). Case 5.4 about child abuse in Denmark highlights differences in approach between teachers and social professionals in a context where multi-professional working is expected to be the norm.

One of the problems of education systems at the tertiary level is that students are often not provided with the opportunity to learn outside their confined single-disciplinary silos. Social work students rarely have the opportunity to experience inter-professional education with fellow students from psychology or nursing, even though after graduation they will more than likely be working alongside colleagues from different disciplines in their places of work. Bronstein (2003) suggests that the time is right to explore the development of new models and frameworks related to inter-professional work, in recognition of the fact that the creation of cultures of collaboration does not happen without intentional discussion between and amongst professional groups. An increased commitment to inter-professional learning and working seems to be growing in momentum, particularly in the UK, and to a lesser extent in countries like Australia.

Promoting courage in professional life

The regulation of social work practice has traditionally been difficult to achieve, which has resulted in many countries establishing complex licensing and registration arrangements (e.g., the USA, Britain, New Zealand), and others opting (despite continuing pressure on government) for continued self-regulation (Australia). Arguably, people working as professional social workers are 'charged with the responsibility of bringing to public notice the values, attitudes, behaviours and social structures and economic imperatives that cause or contribute to the oppression of human welfare and rights' (Chenoweth and McAuliffe 2008: 13). Hence it is common for codes of ethics to promote as an ethical responsibility the duty of social workers to take appropriate action if they consider that a colleague has acted unethically. Many social workers witness activities and behaviours of colleagues that cause harm to vulnerable clients, yet often there is a fear of causing upset in a workplace by notifying relevant authorities (Reamer 2006). It takes a certain amount of courage to decide to 'blow the whistle' and report perceived wrongdoing. Again, organisational cultures that uphold ethical practice and support staff who do disclose situations of unethical conduct are those that are more likely to be operating from a sound value position. Manning (2003) in her work on ethical leadership, describes organisations that cultivate either a 'freedom to comment' culture or a 'spiral of silence' culture. In workplaces where practitioners trust others to listen to their views and respect differences of opinion, it is more likely that problems will be openly aired. In organisations where there is mistrust and fear of reprisal should anyone speak out, the culture will be more one of closing down those issues that should be open for discussion. It is clear to see from these descriptions the difference between a healthy organisational culture and one that is not so healthy. The cases in this chapter clearly illustrate what can happen when communication breaks down within organisations, when there is an absence of trusting collegial relationships, and when the organisation is bound to laws or policies that do not uphold what are known to be core values of social work.

References

Banks, S. (2004) *Ethics, Accountability and the Social Professions*, New York: Palgrave Macmillan.

Banks, S. with others (2010) 'Inter-professional ethics: a developing field. Notes from the *Ethics and Social Welfare* Conference, Sheffield, UK, May 2010', *Ethics and Social Welfare*, 4(3): 280–294.

Brody, R. (2005) *Effectively Managing Human Service Organisations*, 3rd edition, Thousand Oaks, CA: Sage Publications.

Bronstein, L. (2003) 'A model for interdisciplinary collaboration', *Social Work*, 48(1): 297–303.

Chenoweth, L. and McAuliffe, D. (2008) *The Road to Social Work and Human Service Practice*, 2nd edition, South Melbourne: Cengage.

McAuliffe, D. (2010) 'Ethical decision-making', in M. Gray and S. Webb (eds) *Ethics and Value Perspectives in Social Work*, New York: Palgrave Macmillan.

Manning, S. (2003) *Ethical Leadership in Human Services: A Multidimensional Approach*, Boston: Allyn & Bacon.

Reamer, F. (2006) *Social Work Values and Ethics*, 3rd edition, New York: Columbia University Press.

Reel, K. and Hutchings, S. (2007) 'Being part of a team: inter-professional care', in G. Hawley (ed.) *Ethics in Clinical Practice: An Inter-professional Approach*, Harlow: Pearson Education.

Case 5.1   Establishing the facts: issues for organisations working with young women in Iran

Introduction

This case is about four young women who absconded from a residential support centre in an Iranian city and how their case was investigated by a social worker based in a crisis intervention station (CIS) on their return. Young women in Iran are constrained in their ways of behaving and communicating within society on the basis of what is called *Islamic Jurisprudence*. Furthermore, the traditional views on the roles of men and women do not allow girls to be as free as boys. They have to respect the law of *Hijaab*, which forbids the appearance of women in public without the whole of the body being covered, except for the palm and around the face – although this may vary a little from place to place. In addition, being friendly with a person of the opposite sex carries a strong risk of prosecution. In these circumstances, working with girls requires a very sensitive manner. A social worker needs to consider the social and familial limitations within which the girls have to live, and to avoid behaving in the very controlling way that families and society often do. Social workers are expected to gain the trust of female clients.

The case

Four girls (one aged 12 years, two aged 15 years, and one aged 16 years) escaped from a young women's support centre and stayed away without permission for several days. This kind of centre is run by the government and provides full-time residential accommodation for orphan girls or those who have been removed from poorly functioning families. The girls stay there until they reach a certain age (usually 18 years old) and after that age they are normally discharged to be independent. The girls' absence was against the rules of the centre. The rules say that clients must not leave the yard of the centre unless the member of staff on duty gives permission (the staff member might or might not be a social worker). These four girls decided to break the rules, so they went out and their absence caused the staff to raise the alarm.

When the girls returned, they were not allowed to enter the residential centre and the member of staff on duty called Line 123, the Social Emergency Service, to pick them up. The Social Emergency Service is an on-call governmental service with a team of helpers, including a social worker and a psychologist, that helps socially troubled people who are in crisis. This service intervenes particularly in cases of child and wife abuse and suicide. The 123 team delivered the girls to a CIS. There are different numbers of CISs in each province in Iran; the number depends on the size and rate of social problems in the cities. All types of urgent cases are brought to these stations until a full plan of action can be implemented. CISs also have some rooms where women in crisis can stay from three to 20 days, so that social workers can find a good way to solve their problems – which might include returning them to their families if possible or sending them to related residential centres.

A female social worker from the CIS undertook an investigation into the circumstances of the girls' absence from the residential centre. When asked to reveal where they had been staying during their absence, the girls insisted that they had been in a religious holy shrine (*Imam zaadeh*). However, the social worker did not believe their account. To discover the facts about where they had been, and who they had spent time with, the social worker sent another female client, as a spy, to the room the girls were occupying in the CIS to see if she could find out more information about what they had been doing. That girl was a former client of the same residential centre the girls had come from and they knew her. So they talked to her about what they had been doing during their absence. The spy learnt that the girls had journeyed to the north of Iran accompanied by their boyfriends. At this point it is necessary to mention that the laws in Iran are strongly intermingled with Islamic principles and because of that, having a boy/girlfriend *per se* is against the law. According to the law, a handshake with a person of the opposite sex or just being under the same roof, either in a room or in a car, is regarded (for both men and women) as a crime. Therefore, the girls would be doubly guilty and it might severely jeopardise their future if the whole story was reported. But the social worker carried on regardless. Although there is no clear instruction for workers of CISs to dig up the truth about clients' activities by force, having correct historical information about clients can help social workers to make a good decision and treatment plan.

The social worker wrote a report based upon the information the spy obtained. Before putting it in the file and giving it to the manager of the CIS, she showed it to the girls to threaten them to acknowledge more details. When the manager of the CIS was informed, she strongly criticised the social worker for the way she gained the information. The manager believed that this method might prevent a fair and correct judgement being made about this case. As a matter or course, the social worker should have begun a friendly professional relationship with the clients so that they could trust her, then, with no compulsion, she should have gathered and presented the sort of information that was required for the situation.

Commentary 1

HABIB AGHABAKHSHI AND ABBAS ALI YAZDANI

This case gives an account of the treatment of four young women in government-run social service organisations in Iran. Before considering the ethical issues involved in the case, it is important to explain how organisations such as the residential support centre and the crisis intervention station are managed and the role social workers play in them.

The role of social workers in residential centres and crisis intervention stations in Iran

Residential centres for children and young people have three roles: support, control and education. In each centre there are three kinds of staff: a manager (more often than not a social worker); social workers; and childcare trainers who work directly with the children and young people. The most important contribution towards bringing up the children is shouldered by the trainers. Trainers are not necessarily academically educated and may not have studied courses related to the helping professions. However, they usually take some on-the-job training courses.

Social workers often supervise the trainers, to see how they treat the young people, what they teach and what reward and punishment systems they apply. Since social workers do not work very closely with children, as the trainers do, the children expect social workers to be trustworthy and confident people, whose authority allows them to ensure that the children's rights are respected. Social workers have more of a supportive role than a controlling role in the centres. Trainers refer children and young people to social workers when they need support and the professional social worker might make an assessment of needs. This role might change to one of mediator in relation to dealings with people and agencies outside the centre. In dealing with external affairs, social workers undertake home visits, speak with judges in the context of court hearings, assess the readiness of children and their parents or family members to meet each other, get involved in solving school-related problems and provide the resources the young people need.

These residential centres have a number of limitations, however. They tend to operate very strict disciplinary procedures and restrictive rules. By law, residential centres have to follow Islamic orders as well as the official rules determined and prescribed by the state. In terms of social or cultural pathology, in developing societies girls are regarded as much more vulnerable than boys. In the case of girls who are socially damaged, this is further intensified. Therefore, it becomes very important that an empowerment approach is adopted in working with girls and young women. Although many procedures are carried out to help boys and girls become self-confident, nevertheless many social concepts like mutual trust, respect towards people as a civil obligation, and a sense of belonging to a group and society are not well taught.

When the rules enforce constraint and overemphasise conformity, adolescents (especially young women) tend to resist the restrictive rules of the centres. Sometimes resistance leads to tough responses from the trainers in order to punish the young women. Typical punishments for everyday misbehaviour might include: making the child stand in a corner facing a wall; refusing permission to watch the television; or forbidding a young woman to play with others. In the case of serious misbehaviour, various forms of physical punishment may be used, ranging from light to severe, although this is rare. An important point to note is that punishment is often preferred to encouragement. It is not recognised that sometimes a small reward to a young woman may result in a big miracle.

Despite the rather limited role social workers take in the residential centres, in the crisis intervention stations they are legally expected to undertake many significant functions. They take part in virtually the whole helping process, from diagnosis to discharge and follow-up work. So they are aware of, and can more easily intervene to improve, the way service users are treated. Most social workers who work in CISs are women. They usually initiate a good professional relationship with the young women and attempt to work towards a situation where the girls are persuaded to return to their families or are able to choose other suitable alternatives. However, a kind of latent fear or lack of trust always exists in girls who have experienced very bad living conditions. It requires the skill of a professional helper to recreate a sense of trust with these young women.

Issues in this case

In this case, it appears that the social worker based in the crisis intervention station was not confident enough to rely on her social work knowledge, so instead she engaged a spy. Where the spy is friend or room-mate, the girls' already weak personalities will become even more damaged through this use of deception. A qualified and experienced social worker might be expected to make an assessment that these girls need to improve their personalities through mutual respect and trust. However, this did not happen in this case.

This case raises the question of when, if ever, it is justified to use deception to gain information in social work. Certainly in this case it was not justified, as the benefits that might be achieved were not sufficient (there was no emergency and no lives were at risk). Indeed, the response of the manager of the CIS was that this approach was not acceptable or useful. Arguably, deception should never be used in this way by social workers, as it undermines the very essence of the social work role. In our view (from our perspectives as a university teacher involved in social work education and a practising social worker), the social worker in this case could have obtained honest information from the girls through developing a friendly and professional relationship and also through being patient.

However, in organisational contexts where the social work role in developing trusting and supportive relationships is not understood or valued, and where the dominant ethos is one of control rather than empowerment, it is easy to see how an organisational ethics based on treating people as objects to be punished and reformed can allow for deception to be regarded as acceptable. If staff members threaten girls instead of helping them, trying to see the best in them and developing mutual trust, then we face a vicious cycle. It is important for qualified social workers to try to change the prevailing ethos in these organisations – starting with the staff members and gradually enabling them to change their approach and behaviour. Social workers need to continue to work towards encouraging the replacement of punishment and insult with loyalty, respect and integrity. This is difficult to establish when the manager is not a professional social worker. However, the role of the managers and staff in developing an ethical organisation is very significant.

Dr Habib Aghabakhshi is Associate Professor at Azaad University, Rudehen, Tehran. He has a Ph.D. in sociology and a Bachelor's degree in social work. He was one of the first students of social work in Iran under Sattareh Farman Farmaian, who established the social work profession in Iran.

Abbas Ali Yazdani, MSW, works in Raha Social Work Clinic in Tehran as a social worker. He also has experience of working in a residential centre for young boys.

Commentary 2

BEVERLEY BURKE

Introduction: reflexivity and anti-oppressive practice

My interpretation of and responses to the actions of the various players in this situation are influenced by my particular social identity, my partial and Westernised knowledge of Iran and my social work practice experiences. Criticism, therefore, can be made of the ethical stance I bring to my analysis of this situation, which is informed by a critical understanding of European philosophical traditions and my commitment to anti-oppressive values in relation to matters of difference, power and inequality.

The case

Within Iran, as in many other countries, practitioners are involved in controlling practices, manipulating power and authority and rationing resources as well as engaging in practices that are ethical, supportive and enabling. Being open, honest and truthful, and acting with integrity within challenging social situations is an important aspect of ethical practice. However, these ethical principles have been ignored, compromised and dismissed by this particular social worker. Developing the conditions for sensitive and effective working with vulnerable young women, and in this case young women who are very aware of the consequences of their actions, is difficult and requires time, patience and skill. It also requires the worker to actively consider how values, social difference and power will affect interactions not only between the young women, but also the individual and collective reactions of the young women towards the worker. However, for reasons that are not made clear in the scenario, the possibility of working in partnership with these young women and listening to their experiences could not be facilitated ethically by this worker.

To gain a better understanding of the situation we need to know how far the worker was able to take into account the young women's perspectives, rights, concerns and values within her practice. Equally we have to consider how the young women understood the role and responsibilities of the worker. Was it ever going to be possible for the young women truthfully to engage with a worker whom they viewed as having particular personal, professional and organisational power? Individually the young women will be very aware of the consequences of their self-determining action and may well have made a conscious decision not to provide certain information, which they believe would result in particular actions being taken against them. Withholding information is one of the means by which the young women can assert the limited power that they have to protect their best interests. The worker should be reflexively mindful of the social, religious and familial pressures to which these young girls are subject. This understanding needs to be assessed in relation to the fact that the young women are vulnerable and are in the care of a residential support centre. The worker morally as well as professionally has a duty of care to ensure that her relationships with the young women do not replicate and reinforce the very situations from which they have been removed.

The worker's failure to fully appreciate how issues of power and inequality shape personal, social and professional relationships leads her not only to consider obtaining information through the use of a 'spy', but also to contemplate that information so obtained can be legitimately used as the basis for developing an assessment that will underpin future practice. In this action not only are the young women's rights abused and professional ethical and practice codes broken, but the involvement of someone else in the deception is also of concern. Did the worker systematically think through the consequences of her action, not only for herself, but also for the 'spy'? Were issues of confidentiality considered? The worker, in her desire to obtain the 'truth' from the young women, has failed to engage in ethical practice, informed by humanistic and social justice values.

Even though Iran has not signed up to the ethics statement of the International Federation of Social Workers and International Association of Schools of Social Work (IFSW and IASSW 2004) the worker has, in my opinion, failed to act as an accountable member of a profession which is guided by globally agreed ethical standards. There is evidence in the case study to suggest that there is an expectation on social workers to gain the trust of those with whom they work and that information should not be obtained through compulsion. The possibilities of engaging in right action in relation to the young women and ensuring that their needs are met can be realised by the manager, who has to have the courage to act. She clearly sees the action of the worker as wrong, and has voiced her concerns. However, noting concern is one thing, action is what is required. Does the manager have the personal power to take action? Will she use the power that she has as a manager to make right a wrong? Or is she subject to other powers or conditions which may make her fail to act?

The organisational context

The manager is not only accountable to the organisation, which employs her, but she has a professional responsibility in relation to maintaining standards of practice. She can use her relative power and influence to co-operate with, or to resist, organisational procedures, customs and cultures. The end result of her actions may or may not produce a conducive context for ethical action – that is, an 'ethically competent organisation'. However, in her condemnation of this particular worker's practice, she has identified herself as someone who is willing to challenge oppressive practice.

Issues of justice also appear to be complicated in this scenario. The young women initially failed to tell the truth to the worker, who, picking up on this, decided to use another method to obtain the truth of the situation. We also have to look at issues of fairness in relation to the worker – has she up until this point worked ethically? How seriously does the organisation view this breach of practice? The manager needs to be conscious of the range of ethical practice complications that the worker's action has presented to her and take action that is fair and just. This will not be easy, as she has to reflect on her position as a manager – how far, for example, has she provided conditions within supervision for the worker to discuss her practice issues and develop ethical practice? The manager needs to ensure that her approach enables her to hear and understand the ethical reasoning presented by the worker for the actions taken. She also has to ensure that the service users are supported. This is not an easy task – weighing up issues of justice, care, autonomy and integrity will require a full and sensitive discussion with all involved. Finally, she has to take into account the expectations of the agency, the organisational rules and the organisation's reputation and effectiveness.

Conclusions

Wider economic, political, legal and religious systems set particular boundaries with which organisations have to contend. How far an organisation promotes ethical practice is dependent on how the organisational internal systems, policies and cultures are supportive of developing an environment where it is possible to engage in discussions around values and ethics. This requires a culture where codes of ethics and practice are dynamic documents, which are not used to support defensive practices, but are used in conjunction with other strategies to develop and sustain ethical practice. Commitment to change practices requires courage and a preparedness to challenge. The manager in this scenario has a pivotal role to play in the process of further developing and sustaining ethical practice.

Reference

International Federation of Social Workers and International Schools of Social Work (2004) *Ethics in Social Work, Statement of Principles*, IFSW and IASSW.

Beverley Burke is a Senior Lecturer in Social Work at Liverpool John Moores University, United Kingdom. She has practised as a social worker in the field of child care, has published in the area of anti-oppressive practice and is a co-editor of the practice section of the journal, *Ethics and Social Welfare*.

Questions for discussion about Case 5.1

1 Are there any occasions when you think it might be ethically acceptable to use deception in social work?
2 Given the cultural and religious context of social work in Iran, to what extent do you think social workers can develop 'empowering practice' with young women? What would empowering practice look like and how would social workers achieve it in practice?
3 What do you think counts as an 'ethical organisation'? Might the concept of an 'ethical organisation' be different in different practice settings and in different countries?

Case study 5.2

Case 5.2 Deciding on the right to health care insurance: a case from Peru

Introduction

This case comes from Peru and is narrated by a postgraduate student social worker. After finishing her degree, she had been working as a social worker for eight years and at that time she was one of the social workers employed in the administrative offices of the SIS (*Seguro Integral de Salud*, or Integrated Health Insurance). The SIS was created by law in 2002 as a decentralised public body responsible for administering government funds allocated for health care for people who are extremely poor and have no other form of health insurance. Social workers are employed in the operations management section of the SIS, in the 'affiliations area' (*area de afiliaciones*), which is responsible for formulating and implementing standards in relation to the identification and affiliation of SIS users. Among its tasks, this area is in charge of coordinating the staff of the health establishments at the national level in order to ensure the fulfilment of the standards allowing access to health insurance, as well as resolving as a last resort those cases that are not clearly defined by the legislation due to their specific characteristics.

The case

I was working in the affiliations area of the management of operations section of the SIS in a town in Peru. Three social workers work in this area. One of them is in charge of coordination, with administrative support staff. Being a technical area, according to the institutional internal regulation, the staff should not engage with the public directly. However, since this area of work was created and due to the demand from members of the public to solve their problems, the affiliations area has developed an internal policy of dealing directly with individuals and undertaking problem-solving, which is now part of its function.

One day, a woman came to the operations management section of the SIS with her three-year-old son. The child was not in an emergency situation, but needed specialised outpatient care. The woman was really angry because she had taken her son to the Child Health Institute and the staff had refused to take care of him. The reason given was that the admissions staff of that Institute had discovered that the boy's father was covered by social security insurance. The mother told the admissions officer that the father had never recognised his children and that she had not had any contact with him for several years. She had not initiated a process in order to claim for maintenance of their children, nor for social security insurance.

It should be noted at this point that the insurance provided by the SIS is intended for people who are in poverty and do not have any other health insurance, private or public. These requirements are included in a Supreme Decree as well as in several Ministry Resolutions. The law on social security also states that all fathers or mothers entitled to this insurance may also include their children under 18 years old in the coverage. This is the reason why admissions staff in health centres, before agreeing to take care of a child in the framework of the SIS, check whether either of the parents holds another kind of health insurance. As in many countries, abandonment by fathers is quite frequent, mainly in the poorest social layers; in those cases, the mothers take all responsibility for their children. As a result, children often suffer as a result of their fathers' lack of responsibility.

In this case, a conflict arose for me: I had to decide whether the three-year-old child was entitled to the SIS. On the one hand, there were institutional standards and regulations establishing the requirements needed for access to this system, which indicated that this child was not eligible. On the other hand, I was faced with the real situation of this child – his father had not recognised him – so even though he might be entitled to the coverage provided by his father's social security, he could not enjoy this right because of this lack of recognition.

This dilemma particularly challenged my actual, effective role as a social worker, my ethical performance, as well as my assessment of the case. It struck at the heart of my professional identity as a social worker, and raised issues about the relationship between professional and public responsibilities. If I decided that the child was entitled to the SIS, this would be against the institutional rules and against the establishment. If I decided otherwise, I would go against the most important principles according to my analysis as a social worker, including the child's right to health.

However, if we examine the institutional rule for eligibility for SIS, it does not actually take into account a number of social situations, such as parental abandonment, as was the case with this family. This is detrimental not only to this child, but to many others as well, according to the statistics about cases similar to this that I and other colleagues have been collecting.

So, faced with this dilemma, my decision, and that of my colleagues, was to give priority to the child's right to health, and also the 'best interests of the child' as defined in the International Convention for the Rights of the Child, which Peru has signed and ratified. The country's Code for Children and Teenagers also includes this protection measure. Taking these factors into account, we felt we had to take the decision of granting the SIS to this child.

The SIS is a public entity with different hierarchical levels. Therefore, although we had decision-making power in some social cases, we also had to ask for and obtain the manager's consent. This managerial position carries a high turnover rate, so every time we found ourselves facing a similar case we had to explain the problem again to a new person. In this case, we had to explain to the manager the link between national and international legislation and the potential legal action that these families could file with the Ministry of Health due to the lack of care for their children. Finally, the manager supported our decision and we got his permission.

But we also wanted to grant the SIS to all other children with a similar problem. Social workers in the affiliations section had to coordinate the affiliations policy with all the staff in the health centres from the Ministry of Health. Thus we had to coordinate with other social workers who did not belong to the SIS staff, but who work in other health-related institutions, so they could advise the mothers to start legal proceedings in order to achieve recognition and maintenance, since this was also their children's right.

My final comments on this case are as follows. While working with and for people as social workers, especially in such a vital field as health, the practical lesson is that we will have to confront many dilemmas. However, the most important point is to know how to confront them, including knowing that we can use many tools without breaking the professional code of ethics. Above all, a fundamental principle is that of human solidarity, which is an important reference point for me and has helped me a lot in my job: 'treat others as you would like them to treat you'.

Taking decisions is not an easy task, and this is even more true in the field of social work, where day after day we (the professionals) have to identify human and social problems of great complexity. So I believe it is important to have a series of theoretical and practical tools, such as the ones we have learned throughout our ethics in social work course, that help us to improve our interventions and, above all, to act without betraying our principles and values as caring professionals.

Commentary 1

MARÍA JESÚS ÚRIZ PEMÁN

Background on Peru

To understand the issues involved in this case, we need to understand the economic and social conditions of the country in which it takes place. In Peru, 51% of the population is considered to be poor and 30% to be living in extreme poverty. The situation of Peruvian people as regards health is directly linked to their socio-economic condition. Health problems have several causes, mainly derived from poverty and social exclusion.

Poverty levels and their expressions are not the same throughout the country. There is an average of 25% of children suffering from chronic malnutrition. Furthermore, 72% of children under two years of age suffer from anaemia due to a lack of micronutrients. It has been proved that social policies directed at children do not reach all those for whom they are intended, and that the leakage levels of grants are very high.

The right to health involves an adequate, continuing and deliberate progress of public policies, as well as the allocation of budgets and an effective impact on the communities' health levels. The budget assigned in Peru to health is 4.7% of GDP, far from the average of Latin American countries (7.5%).

During the last 25 years, all governments have tried to combat extreme poverty with a number of social programmes of palliative character. The creation of the Integrated Health Insurance (SIS) forms part of the financial reform of the Ministry of Health, whose fundamental aim is to reduce the economic barriers that limit the poor population's access to health services, unprotected by the social security system, as well as the implementation of new payment methods to providers of health services. This system is thus the most important instrument for the achievement of universal coverage.

Ethical issues

Reinterpreting institutional rules and promoting the creation of other standards

This case illustrates the dilemma of a social worker between prioritising the right of a child to health or strictly following an institutional rule. Strictly speaking, interpreting the institutional rules in a literal way, this child was eligible for health coverage under the National Health Insurance (through his father), and not to the coverage under the SIS. However, this strict application of the rules would have meant that the child would have been excluded from health care coverage (as there was no contact with the father), thus violating his fundamental right to health care. This case is a clear example of how institutional rules are sometimes too narrow or fail to cover real situations of great need. It is time to try to change those rules to accommodate these new real situations. But how do these changes occur?

One could note in this case that the role of social workers is not limited to mechanically applying the established rules, but also to reinterpreting and trying to modify a rule when they perceive it is not really providing an answer to the user's needs. Nowadays, with the bureaucratisation of work, the role of many social professionals (and also social workers) as mere 'social controllers' (who must control which users are eligible to access to a particular service) or 'service providers' is subject to strong criticism. However, situations like the one described here help us to think about a non-bureaucratic and responsive social work. The role of these social workers is so important that they can even reinterpret an institutional rule and promote the creation of a new regulation at the national level.

While Peru has not yet adopted a Ministerial Resolution to govern these kinds of situations, the answer provided in this case and others can form the first steps to a new regulation, which would prevent people in need having to reach the last level of the health care system in order to solve a problem that could have been addressed at their primary health care centre.

Direct contact with users

The social worker involved in this case referred to the principle of human solidarity and the role of the professional code of ethics. Social workers are often the professionals who have the most direct contact with users and, therefore, those who have the most direct knowledge about their needs. Furthermore, this privileged position allows them to identify the limitations and implementation difficulties of many regulations. They can therefore play an active role in the development and evolution of institutional rules, ensuring their effectiveness and ensuring that they provide a real answer to people in need.

The role played by codes of ethics

Today, some people dispute the meaning and purpose of professional codes of ethics. Some think codes are just abstract documents full of platitudes and therefore meaningless. In this case, however, the view of this social worker as regards her code of ethics has an immediate, practical application; it makes her prioritise the people in need and especially the disadvantaged people, such as that child.

My opinion in this particular case is that social workers have an important role to play in developing organisations. They have to be confident in themselves and not be afraid to propose institutional changes. They are often in a privileged position to detect the inefficiency of some procedures and to propose new challenges to improve the quality of organisations and to support people who need help.

María Jesús Úriz Pemán, Ph.D., is Professor of Philosophy in the social work department at the Public University of Navarre, Spain.

Commentary 2

LYNNE M. HEALY

This case illustrates the conflicting ethical and practice obligations of the social worker. Elements of equality, harm and duty to follow agency rules and laws are involved. By citing the United Nations Convention on the Rights of the Child, the social worker brings human rights principles to the forefront in considering the case.

Social work practice in many nations is increasingly governed by regulations and bureaucratic procedures. An excessive emphasis on efficiency and cost reduction may override client needs and curb the ability of social workers to respond ethically to practice situations. In this case, the social workers have resisted bureaucratic rules. Although regulations state that social workers in the administrative office should not engage with the public, the staff has developed its own procedures and does in fact assist individuals with their problems. Inevitably, additional dilemmas for the social workers arise, as individual situations do not fit neatly into agency regulations.

In analysing the ethical decisions made in this case, it is significant that the child's situation is not an emergency. The author indicates that although the child needs special medical care, the situation does not require immediate attention. Therefore, there is no threat of immediate physical harm to the child, allowing the social worker time to consider the impact of her decision on the child, the parent(s), the decision climate within the agency and the availability of resources for potentially more needy clients in the future.

Human rights and ethical decision-making

In resolving the case and deciding to grant an exception to the policy, the social worker cites the United Nations Convention on the Rights of the Child (CRC) (1989). Human rights principles are highly relevant to social work theory, practice and ethics. The SIS social worker notes that the Convention includes a child's right to health care; the fact that Peru has ratified the treaty and therefore committed the country to bringing its laws and practices into compliance is an important justification for extending health insurance to the client in the case. However, much like social work ethics, human rights principles can come into conflict with each other and do not therefore provide easy resolution of ethical dilemmas.

In Article 3 (1), the CRC emphasises the concept of the best interests of the child: 'In all actions concerning children, whether undertaken by public or private social welfare institutions, courts of law, administrative authorities or legislative bodies, the best interests of the child shall be a primary consideration.' The challenge for the social worker is to determine 'best interests'.

The CRC does indeed very explicitly include the right to health care. Article 24 (1) specifies that: 'States Parties recognize the right of the child to the enjoyment of the highest attainable standard of health and to facilities for the treatment of illness and rehabilitation of health. States Parties shall strive to ensure that no child is deprived of his or her right of access to such health care services.' This clearly supports the decision of the social worker to extend health coverage to the client in the case and the obligations of the government to provide access.

But the treaty also guarantees children the right to be acknowledged by their parents, a right that may be undermined by the case decision. Article 7 requires that all children be registered at birth and includes 'the right to know and be cared for by his or her parents'. The Convention further requires States to ensure that the right to know one's parents is realised: 'States Parties shall use their best efforts to ensure recognition of the principle that both parents have common responsibilities for the upbringing and development of the child' (Article 18). Thus, more emphasis on fathers' responsibilities is an essential component to safeguarding children's rights. It is possible that by covering the child under the SIS, the mother will be less motivated to contact the child's father.

Utilitarian approaches to ethics

In granting SIS coverage to children who may be entitled to other insurance, scarce resources may be diverted from more needy cases. The utilitarian approach to ethical decision-making is based on evaluation of the consequences or the 'goodness' of the outcome. Utilitarian analysis can be based on the 'act' or the 'rule' (Reamer 2000; see also Chapter 4 in this book). The decision made by the social worker in this case satisfies the conditions of act utilitarianism, meaning that the social worker chose the optimal outcome for the individual. In rule utilitarianism, the social worker or manager must consider the consequences if the same decision were to be made in all cases. Thus, in this case, covering children who do not meet eligibility requirements might exhaust the resources of the SIS. Wise and careful use of resources is recognised as an ethical responsibility in some social work ethical codes. The United States code of social work ethics specifically states that 'social workers should be diligent stewards of the resources of employing organizations, wisely conserving funds where appropriate' (NASW 2008: 3.09g). Applying rule utilitarianism might have resulted in a different case decision.

Finally, ethical decisions involving children are particularly difficult, as their rights are inevitably entangled with the rights of adults, especially parents. Children pay for the consequences of adults' decisions and actions. In this case, the child is suffering from the father's lack of responsibility and acknowledgement and possibly from the mother's reluctance to pursue the father. The social worker should therefore investigate ways to encourage the father to accept his paternal responsibilities, unless the relationship would pose a danger to the child. In the meantime, the social worker's decision has ensured that the child will receive the necessary medical care.

References

NASW (2008) *Code of Ethics*, Washington, DC: National Association of Social Workers.

Reamer, F. (2000) 'Administrative ethics', in R. Patti (ed.), *Handbook of Social Welfare Management*, Thousand Oaks, CA: Sage.

United Nations (1989) *Convention on the Rights of the Child*, www.ohchr. org, accessed November, 2010.

Lynne M. Healy, MSW, Ph.D., is Professor and Director, Center for International Social Work Studies, University of Connecticut, West Hartford, Connecticut, USA. She has lived her whole life in the New England area of the United States, although extensively involved in intercultural and international work and travel.

Questions for discussion about Case 5.2

1 This case shows how social workers resist playing the role of bureaucrats (simply following existing rules), partly justifying this with reference to children's rights. In what ways are the human rights principles raised by the case author helpful in making ethical decisions? How would you compare this case of 'acting outside the regulations' with Case 5.4 about 'bending the law' in relation to child protection in Denmark?

2 The social worker in this case said it 'struck to the heart of my professional identity as a social worker'. What do you think she means by this? How important is a strong 'professional identity' in contexts where social workers are striving for organisational change?

3 This case shows how laws and policies for the distribution of state-funded benefits to poor people may exclude those in real need. What might be the implications if the rules were changed so that it was easier for single mothers to claim benefits for their children in cases where the fathers will not take responsibility or cannot be traced? What happens in your own country?

Case study 5.3

Case 5.3   The vicious cycle: issues for a church-based social worker in Australia

Introduction

The following account is written in the first person by an Australian social worker (male) based on his professional and personal experiences. The case relates to the support offered by a church-based counselling service to a young man with schizophrenia. The Australian mental health system includes a government network of community-based and hospital services, which usually employ social workers and mental health nurses to deliver individualised casework support. Agencies in the community also receive funding for individual and family support programmes (including counselling) like the one described in the scenario. Large church networks form a significant proportion of the social services infrastructure in

Australia, especially in the southern states. Their services are usually funded by the state but issues of ideology and motivation frequently arise.

The case

I stared at the phone and groaned. I had just spent more than 45 minutes in a long and heated discussion with a caseworker from the Community Mental Health Service, who seemed like a good guy but . . . well, he could get very *passionate* about his work.

Things were not going according to plan. For years, I had worked for a few hours each week as a volunteer in my church's counselling service while I completed my social work degree. I had always felt that the church, and the counselling service, could make a real difference in the local community – a place which was, in my experience, both materially and spiritually impoverished. I should know – I grew up there.

Over the last year I had worked hard to secure funding for the service from a government grant. I prepared submissions, and sought the support of the church board so that the service could be properly funded with a professional coordinator and housed in a shopfront in a local mall. It was with a mix of pride and trepidation that I then accepted the position as coordinator of the service. It seemed like the culmination of all of my dreams that my professional, personal and spiritual values could come together to really make a difference.

The man on the phone was the caseworker for Spiro, a member of the church and a client of the counselling service. Spiro was a troubled and brooding young man who would attend church and youth programmes diligently for months, and participate enthusiastically in church activities and services – then disappear from the face of the earth, only to resurface a month or so later. As far as I could recall, this pattern was established over a couple of years.

Now I knew why. The caseworker had informed me that Spiro had schizophrenia, and, during his worst times, Spiro was unable to function in the mainstream community. He was prone to intrusive delusions and crippling paranoia, and, when he was unwell, he would usually sit alone in his tiny unit staring at the walls until a neighbour or family member arranged for him to be admitted to hospital. Over the last few years, his 'episodes', hospitalisation and treatment had fallen into a predictable cycle.

In hospital, Spiro was responsive and insightful. The hospital staff would assist him in understanding his illness and maintaining compliance with treatment (both medication and regular psychotherapy). Balanced, settled and strong, Spiro would be discharged from hospital.

Within a few weeks Spiro would resume his friendships, supported employment and social activities. The central pillar of his social world was the church community. Once he returned to church (looking well and coping well), he would start attending counselling with the church counselling service, seeing the same counsellor – Arthur, an elder from the church – each time.

Arthur was a likeable, sociable man in his 60s who was one of the members of the church board. He had supported the submission for funding for the counselling service and had personally encouraged me to apply for the coordinator's position.

According to the caseworker, Arthur would, with disturbing predictability, counsel and support Spiro to go off his medication. With faith, support and the grace of God, Arthur maintained, Spiro could overcome his illness and find a way of living free from psychoactive drugs and psychiatrists. Spiro, feeling strong and confident, would invariably follow Arthur's advice.

After a few weeks of 'success', celebrated and encouraged by Arthur and other members of the church, Spiro would start to become unwell. Neither Arthur nor anyone else would see Spiro in the long, lonely days in his empty room, as his mental health deteriorated and his illness asserted itself.

This was when the mental health system would step in to pick up the pieces, to assess Spiro, take him to hospital, and start the cycle again.

Only this time, things had not taken the same course. Spiro, after release from hospital (and in a seemingly lucid and rational state), had made a suicide attempt. He was in hospital again and the hospital was refusing to support any discharge plans until I could guarantee that I would prevent any further contact between Arthur and Spiro. Furthermore, the caseworker was threatening to contact the counselling service's funding bodies and report that the service was ineffective (at best) and downright dangerous (at worst).

I spoke with the pastor of my church and explained what was happening to Spiro, and that this could threaten the credibility of the counselling service. Although he could understand and acknowledge these issues, he took the position that:

1   the approach was consistent with the teaching of the church – faith and hope were central beliefs and Spiro *could* overcome his illness with God's help;
2   I had been employed by the church because I shared their vision for the service and I was expected to implement the values of the church; and

3   Arthur was a church elder who had helped develop the counselling service and who was now the head of its management committee – he had a right to direct the style of service it offered.

All of my great feelings of congruence and purpose quickly dissipated in the face of this clash – I thought I knew what I was doing but I felt like my professional and personal selves were at war.

This experience caused me to look honestly at my own growth over the preceding years, especially at the way that my own values had been challenged, confronted and renegotiated through my university studies. I was starting to see my underpinning religious convictions as the 'raw material' for social work values rather than as an end in themselves or as a set of non-negotiable organising principles. I was, for the first time, struck by what I came to believe was an essential incompatibility between fundamentalist Christian values and effective social work practice (although I acknowledge freely that this is by no means a universal position on the issue). So, resolution was simple but painful – I left the position soon after to start a career in a statutory child protection position.

Commentary 1

TRUUS FRAAIJE, HAN AALBERS AND PETER VAN ZILFHOUT

Into the case

'The vicious cycle' suggests the certainty of a mechanism. In this case, the certainty of imbalance in Spiro's health during his life caused by schizophrenia. The downward spiral is bent upwards every time by neighbours or a family member's intervention. Even after his suicide attempt, the pastor of the church shares the point of view that Spiro can overcome his illness with faith. But in his loneliest moments Spiro has no support. The hospital makes the difference by demanding a guarantee that there is no more contact between Arthur and Spiro. Soon afterwards the social worker who tells us his story left the position to start a new career.

From our point of view, this case presents us with a surprise. In the Netherlands, religion has become more and more an individual orientation. The position presented by Arthur has almost disappeared. We eliminated the role and strength of faith in social work, instead of empowering it. Is it not the government's responsibility to take care of the main human interests in society – especially towards social needs? We left the church with its rules and regulations. But we also left the rituals, the celebrations, the security and the certainty. We see clearly that the service was a shelter for Spiro, but for the social worker it turned out to be stifling. In the end, it seems, Spiro was left alone.

From an organisational point of view we can envision some practical possibilities and solutions, which might include: professionalising Arthur and the whole centre; introduction of planning, control and hierarchy; introduction of scientific knowledge; introduction of supervision; assessing the need for collective values based on professional knowledge.

However, ethical and professional questions will remain. Should dedicated social workers stay in charge in an organisation as depicted in this case? Should the organisation not adjust to the modern world and find answers to questions like: What is our contribution to the community? What new opportunities can we offer? What is our responsibility to society? What is our strength?

We sense a great opportunity in this unbearable and heartbreaking situation. Professional social workers, we think, have to stay where they are and increase their influence. They have to present themselves as professionals in the way of Aristotle's concept, 'phronesis'. With 'phronesis' ('practical wisdom'), they can make a difference. They have to act as able and willing professionals who make the right decisions. But it is not only about acting the right way, it is also about acting for the right reason. This is an important distinction: the different parties do not have to be afraid of losing their identities. Social care, health care, mental care, community care and their scientific foundations, along with religion with its rituals and celebrations, can fulfil people's needs. With respect for each other, it must be possible that each professional can take the responsibility without threatening the other. Our goal is to serve our clients, not an idea.

The case revisited

Often a presentation of a case ends with a question: What to do? What to think? What to wish for? – the so called 'case question'. A case normally starts at a point where the key actor feels a lack of competence about how to handle a given situation professionally and personally. Usually it is this specific feeling (anger, fear/angst, powerlessness, frustration, etc.) that opens up the case, at least when it is taken as a starting point for reflection.

The given case meets these demands: the emotion is there, the story of the case starts with groaning – after 'a long and heated discussion'. And yes, the question of what to do is present, albeit hidden, in the form of 'What should I, the worker, do now?' The answer is that the worker leaves his position and starts another job elsewhere, in the child protection field.

All is understandable if we read this story of a client who does not get the treatment needed for his illness because his counsellor from church believes he can overcome his illness with the help of God. Probably we ourselves would do the same as this social worker did, if we ended up in a comparable situation where we could no longer act professionally and personally. And, yes, of course, Spiro, the client involved here, needs to be treated medically, not religiously – he is obviously ill.

Yet something puzzles us in this story, in the way it is told: the worker tells his story with a kind of moral justice. He tells us his motives, but he does not question them. He takes them for granted, talking about: 'great feelings of congruence and purpose'. He uses strong words too: 'professional and personal selves at war'. For someone for whom his work is 'a culmination of all my dreams that my professional, personal and spiritual values could come together to really make a difference', the story of Spiro, who ends up in hospital after a suicide attempt, could only be frustrating – a disillusion even in this perspective. This means that the case presented here refers not so much to Spiro, rather, the story tells us something about the worker himself in our opinion: his demands, his wishes, his hopes, his motives and his goals are at stake. We sincerely doubt whether this is a case of ethical and professional confrontation only, although we are convinced too that clients and patients need proper treatment and that this should not be withheld from them for religious reasons. Nonetheless, we wonder whether strong hopes, strong determinations and strong convictions for this kind of work – social work – can be too strong? Might there be occasions, like this one, when what is needed is moderation and a time perspective, that is, a more mature and realistic image of the possibilities and impossibilities of social work? People lead their own lives after all, for better or for worse, and we are curious as to whether the social worker could have remained on the job, could have interfered, could have introduced the necessary changes, and at the same time could have become more relaxed about it? Time shows again and again that most cases have an ethical dimension. The 'practical wisdom' of the social workers should lead to a professional attitude that makes these cases more or less solvable, manageable or at least durable.

Ethical principles?

This case presents us with 'the changing of a change-agent'. We sense his excitement at the possibility of uniting different value-systems into a collective whole. Later on, we sense the acceptance of 'growing insight' or of 'loss' in the realisation that in the end it is not possible to unite these value-systems, to unite collective and personal systems, or to confront spiritual truths with professional truths. The case of the social worker shows important changes: he becomes a professional and academic. He also loses faith in the possibilities of ethical congruence in values and in the compatibility between values and effective practice. The social worker ends with trust in his individual grip on values and in professional care for clients.

What can we conclude? One conclusion might be that personal, professional and spiritual values cannot and will not be shared collectively, even in an organisation with colleagues sharing the same ideals. Values are 'raw material' and only in real life do they demonstrate their worth. Another conclusion is that in every ethical dilemma we can discern a professional dilemma as well and perhaps the reverse is also true. We see in this case that the values of the social worker really matter and bear an effect on the future and well-being of a client. Finally, we conclude that when people work in the community in which they grew up, this makes them especially vulnerable.

Truus Fraaije is a pedagogue and philosopher, and lecturer at the Fontys Hogeschool of Social Work, Eindhoven, the Netherlands.
Han Aalbers is a social worker and sociologist, and lecturer at the Fontys Hogeschool of Social Work, Eindhoven, the Netherlands.
Peter van Zilfhout is a philosopher and lecturer at the Fontys Hogeschool of Social Work, Eindhoven, the Netherlands.

Commentary 2

MELISSA FLOYD

The intersection between our worlds of faith and our professional worlds is rife with the potential for ethical conflicts, grey areas and, most basically, those vague feelings of unease. While it is always easier to analyse ethical conflicts from afar than when one is embroiled in them, certain aspects of this case are more troubling than others. Examining each area in turn helps clarify the situation and illuminate possible courses of action.

Dual relationships and role conflict

While 'dual relationships' or relationships where a clinician is also an acquaintance and, in this case, a church member may be unavoidable in rural locations, they are still problematic in that they set up a certain amount of role conflict. When these roles are mutually exclusive – as is the case with a social worker who must adhere to tenets such as 'do no harm', and the role of a church member in a church where medical interventions are frowned upon – the social worker is left with a dilemma.

Multiple organisations with conflicting value systems

The presence of multiple organisations in this case with conflicting value systems makes negotiating ethical concerns even more complex. Hospitals tend to align with the medical model, where medication intervention and expert and patient roles are highlighted. Churches are a diverse group and difficult to categorise, but this particular church seems to endorse a more fundamentalist belief system, which downplays and even negates the need for mental health medication. The social worker, acting as coordinator, needs to advocate both for the client individually, as well as for the continued funding of the counselling centre. Issues of risk management and liability are also prominent here as the centre itself as well as the social worker individually are at great risk of litigation should Spiro harm himself or others when acting on the elder's recommendation to stop his medication. The funding agencies who have granted the counselling centre monies are other organisations involved. The mental health centre where the case manager works also has clear ideas about the perceived mismanaging of Spiro's case. Finally, if the social worker in the case is licensed, the accrediting body may also be involved and the social worker could be at risk of being sanctioned if the accrediting body considered his actions (or non-actions) to be unethical.[1]

'Who is the client and what do they want?'

Analysing who is the client in this case may help to clarify a course of action. Clearly, the client is Spiro; however, less clear are Spiro's own

---

1 In Australia there is no system of licensing of social workers as such, but the Australian Association of Social Workers has a code of ethics and a system for dealing with complaints about unethical conduct.

preferences in this case. The case centres more on the feelings of the confused social worker, the angry caseworker and hospital staff, the crusading elder and the uncompromising pastor. Does Spiro also want to stop his medication or is he being unduly influenced by the elder's beliefs? The suicide attempt may indicate that Spiro is conflicted and depressed about his choices. If we make the client's concerns paramount, then other people's agendas fall behind and the path of best practice becomes more apparent.

So what is best?

Again, it is always easier to direct from afar. However, as I see it this social worker has serious decisions to make. It may be impossible for him to continue simultaneously being a member of this church, serving as the coordinator for the counselling centre and being true to social work mandates of doing no harm. Clearly the suicide attempt mandates quick decision-making, the stakes are now 'life and death'.

This being said, two immediate courses of specific action emerge for the social worker in this case: 1) do nothing (that is, continue to have the elder counsel Spiro into discontinuing his medication) and be in conflict with the mental health system, the hospital and personal and social work values; or 2) refuse to comply with the pastor's directive to support the elder, putting the social worker at risk of losing his job. If the social worker chooses the second course of action, he would probably need to replace the elder on Spiro's case with himself and work to help Spiro reconcile his clear need for ongoing medication with his religious views.

In the United States this same situation would not be uncommon. I am left wondering if the pastor's and elder's views would change if Spiro had, say, diabetes and needed insulin or had cancer and needed chemotherapy? It may be that the church in question stigmatises mental illness as 'sin'. In this case, the social worker could offer to do educational programmes to help with lessening these misconceptions. The situation would be less complex if the social worker were not also a member of the church, since this brings issues of personal history and private life into the professional realm. Continuing to serve in multiple, conflicting roles puts this social worker at risk both emotionally and professionally, as illustrated in this case, and leaves him embroiled in his own 'vicious cycle'.

Melissa Floyd is Associate Professor of Social Work, University of North Carolina, Greensboro, USA.

Questions for discussion about Case 5.3

1   According to the author of the case, churches play a significant role in delivering social services in parts of Australia, and 'issues of ideology and motivation frequently arise'. What safeguards do you think should be put in place to ensure all social services are delivered to acceptable professional standards, especially when volunteers are involved? What is the role of religious organisations in offering social services in your own area/country?

2   This case was complicated by the fact that the social worker was a member of the congregation of the church for which he also worked as a coordinator. What are the advantages and disadvantages of 'dual relationships' and what would you do to mitigate the disadvantages?

3   Apart from leaving his job, what other courses of action do you think might have been available to the social worker? What ethical justifications might be offered for each course of action (including leaving the job)?

Case study 5.4

Case 5.4   Bending the law? A case about reporting child abuse in Denmark

Introduction

This case is about how a school in Denmark responded to children's accounts of violence in their homes. In Denmark it is against the law for parents or professionals to hit children under the age of 18 years old. The Parents' Responsibility Act (1995) states that: 'The child must be treated with respect for its person, and must not be subjected to physical punishment or other abusive treatment.' Through the Social Service Act (1998), the social authorities of the local municipality (which employs social workers) are responsible for the protection of children against abuse, violence or neglect. This covers measures for general prevention as well as for intervention in individual cases of children subjected to abuse or otherwise in need of help and protection.

The Social Service Act also imposes a duty to report about child abuse on 'frontline' professionals working with children, youth and families, i.e., social care workers, community workers, youth workers, teachers and nurses. If they become aware of possible child abuse, child neglect or children in need of help and protection these persons have by law an obligation to report to the local social authorities what they know in order that the child receives the appropriate help. The case that follows was initially reported in an article in the magazine of the Danish teachers' organisation under the headline: 'Teacher shocked about the extent of violence against children.'[2] In an interview, the teacher and the principal of the school recounted how the teacher accidentally became aware of extensive domestic violence towards the children in her class, and how the school dealt with this problem through parents' meetings with information, role plays and dialogue. The story was picked up by a national morning paper and presented on the front page as: 'School failed to report about violence against children.'[3] This initiated an intensive public debate – including contributions from several politicians – about child protection, cultural differences and the professional duty to report about child abuse (*underretningspligten* in Danish).

The case

Maryam E. was the class teacher for children in the second grade (eight-year-olds) in a state school situated in an area of Copenhagen with a majority of first- and second-generation immigrant or refugee families. The families come from many different countries, but large groups are immigrants from Turkey and refugees from Arab countries in the Middle East. Maryam E. herself came to Denmark from Palestine in 1990. In her class she has 24 children of which around 75% have an immigrant or refugee background. After some incidents of bullying and fights among the children, Maryam E. decided to address the theme of violence and conflict management with the class. 'Especially the boys use violence as a way of communicating. Many have a limited vocabulary and easily lose their temper', she said. The challenge for Maryam E. was to help the children to develop better ways to handle conflicts, for instance to speak

2 *Folkeskolen*, February 2009, 'Lærer chokeret over omfanget af vold mod børn' [Teacher shocked about the extent of violence against children].
3 *Politiken*, 5 February 2009, 'Skole undlod at melde vold mod børn' ['School failed to report about violence towards children'], and page 5: 'Vold i hjemmet er et stort dilemma i skolen' ['Violence at home is a big dilemma in the school'].

up instead of fighting back. She asked the children to write a letter to her (using words or pictures) about what kind of conflicts they experienced and how they handled them at home. When Maryam E. saw the letters she was 'shocked'. A majority of the letters (70%) were about violence, about the children being hit. Some of the children experienced being hit with a hard hand; one child had drawn a picture of a coat hanger with which he was hit; and another one, a stick. Some children wrote that their mother was hit.

Maryam E. was painfully aware of her legal obligation as a teacher to report to the social authorities about child abuse, but she did not believe it to be the best way to reach the parents and to change the ways in the families. She discussed the problem with the principal of the school and it was decided to confront the parents of the children in the class as a group in order to establish a dialogue about conflict management in the families. No reports were written to the social authorities. What happened was that the school (the principal, the class teachers and a 'social pedagogical' teacher working with the school's 'problem children') invited the parents to a meeting about how to stop violent conflicts in the class. Almost all parents showed up. Through role plays and group discussions the teachers wanted to establish a dialogue with the parents and to make the point that children learn from their parents how to handle conflict. If parents themselves use or allow violence, then they tell the children through their acts that violence is right. During the meeting the teachers also told the parents about the letters, and about Danish law. Furthermore, they informed the parents about the teachers' duty to report about violence against children. From the dialogue with the parents the school learned that many immigrant and refugee families in that area live in a 'parallel society' and know very little about the Danish society and Danish norms about bringing up children. They have no idea that it is neither allowed nor regarded useful to hit one's children.

The meeting was a success according to the principal and Maryam. Some months later they experienced less bullying and fighting among the children in the class, and the parents became more trustful and open to the teachers about the problems they faced with their children at home.

The reactions

The article provoked much public reaction in the media, and the school was heavily criticised for letting the children down and for not fulfilling their legal obligation to report about child abuse. For example, a politician from the Copenhagen City Council commented that he was shocked about the extent of violence towards children in immigrant families, but even more shocked to learn about the 'irresponsible' reaction of the school: 'Either they don't know the law and their duty to report,' he said 'or they are too afraid to confront the parents.' The head of the Children's Rights Organisation in Denmark put it this way:

> All children have a right not to be hit. Period. That right must not be bent, and neither must the law and the duty of the professionals to report to the social authorities about violence against children. That 70% of the children in a class are hit, does not make the problem less serious for the individual child. It would be a great help for these children to have social authorities and a social worker contact the family to investigate the situation and decide about which measures should be taken in the best interest of the child.

In one of the interviews the principal explained the reasons for the school's choice:

> If we had sent off a whole pile of reports, then five or six families would probably have turned their backs on us, moved their children to a private school run by their own minority ethnic group and continued to beat their children. Many other parents would have thought that those teachers are not to be trusted, and we shall never again tell them about our family life. Instead we had this fantastic meeting with an open and fruitful exchange. I am sure the parents will not continue to beat their children. They will think about it. I know very well what is the law, but I also know what reality is like in the social service department, lacking I don't know how many social workers. We should not be so rigid, that we don't try to handle these problems within the school – instead of leaving 15–16 reports to lie on a table drowned in all kinds of other cases. We are not afraid to confront the problem. On the contrary. It is an easy and comfortable solution for us just to send off the papers to the social service department. The difficult choice for us is to engage in discussion directly with the parents. In my world it is a positive story about how to reach certain parents in alternative ways. I believe we ought to get a medal!

Commentary 1

MARIANNE SKYTTE

This case inspires many different comments. Children's right to protection against abuse is, of course, not a matter of debate. But you can discuss the general dilemma with laws that prohibit certain ways of child rearing. Is this type of law effective in changing the way citizens reflect on their parenthood and act as parents? Or is it more possible that this type of legislation will lead to both professional and parental silencing and denial of the problems some children face in order to avoid sanctions from the child protection authorities? This could happen if the legislation does not create new possibilities for supporting parents' reflections around their child rearing. By focusing on the prohibition and sanctioning of hitting a child, for example, this kind of legislation may itself – contrary to its intentions – become a barrier rather than an engine for developing more respectful child rearing.

In this commentary I shall, however, limit myself to commenting on the problems that can occur when the work of welfare state professionals is influenced by organisational and professional mistrust of each other.

Often professions are presented as knowledge-based groups performing tasks within a certain jurisdiction. But neither the tasks nor the jurisdictions are static units. There is always – though to varying degrees – competition between different professions about jurisdiction over a given task (Abbott 1988; Burrage, Jarausch and Siegrist 1990). Professional competition, or even conflict, between teachers and social workers, both at an individual and at an organisational level, is well known.

In Denmark, we have a long and strong tradition of school–home collaboration. The teachers meet the parents several times a year throughout children's years in elementary school. And often problems around children's everyday life are constructively solved in collaboration between school, parents and the children. The teachers and schools might therefore feel that problems around the well-being of the pupils are best solved by the people involved in the children's everyday lives: the parents and the teachers.

But according to the Danish Social Service Act, teachers who become aware of violence towards children must report this to the local social authorities. To the teachers in this case this is provocative as they, according to the school principal, know that a lack of social workers at the office will result in either no action from the social authorities or a severely delayed action. Against this background the principal and class teacher decide that they had better act themselves, as they are able not only to act now, but also to start a constructive dialogue with the parents.

However, by acting the way they do, the staff at the school do not disclose the situation of the children to the social authorities, who are by law defined as the institution that should handle cases of child abuse. By doing what they themselves think is best for the children, the staff at the school are putting themselves above the existing legislation that has been agreed by the democratically elected parliament. The principal and the teacher are using their professional power to override the democratically determined procedures.

The case illustrates a common challenge for professionals: on the one hand they will use their professional discretion on a daily basis to decide what is best to do; and on the other hand they will also have to recognise that the democratic processes may lead to/have led to another decision about the case at hand. The desire for professional power and for the recognition of professional discretion will often not be in accordance with the desire for a further democratic development of society. While at work, welfare professionals must never break the law; but they should, of course, use their freedom of expression to participate in the debate on the laws!

My opinion about the current case is that the principal of the school could have contacted the head of the district social authorities and told her/him about the situation revealed by the children's letters. The two of them could have had a meeting between themselves, the class teacher Maryam and one or two social workers. Here they could have discussed how to cooperate on the situation. The result of such a meeting could very well have been that the school should start the process by inviting the parents to a meeting, just as they did. At the end of this meeting the head of the social authorities or one of her/his staff could have introduced themselves, their department and their services. By taking action at a level involving all parents and children you could hope to avoid labelling specific parents and children. In this way the school and social authorities could have cooperated in creating a constructive atmosphere for discussing values and norms around child rearing in a social context that seems not yet to be fully known by the migrant parents. And the social authorities could have had a more constructive platform from which to explain why and how they could be contacted by the parents or how and why they themselves were going to contact the parents. In this way the process could have been started off as constructively as the school seems to have wished – without the school violating the law.

References

Abbott, A. (1988) *The System of Professions. An Essay on the Division of Expert Labor*, Chicago and London: The University of Chicago Press.

Burrage, M., Jarausch, K. and Siegrist, H. (1990) 'An actor-based framework for the study of the professions', in M. Burrage and R. Torstendahl (eds), *Professions in Theory and History: Rethinking the Study of the Professions*, London: Sage.

Marianne Skytte is Associate Professor in Social Work at Aalborg University, Denmark. Her research focuses on how the Scandinavian welfare state model and social work practice is challenged by international migrations and the globalised society.

Commentary 2

CHRIS BECKETT

The law in the UK is not identical to that in Denmark, in that it is not illegal to hit children in the UK, provided that the hitting is not of sufficient severity to make a mark. However, as in Denmark, there is an expectation that professionals such as school teachers should refer on any suspicions that children are being maltreated, and this case raises questions that will be very familiar to professionals working with children in the UK. They are questions that go to the very heart of child protection work.

What has happened here is not that the school has ignored the evidence that most of these children are experiencing some sort of violence at home (I assume that in many cases the violence in question will be smacking or beating used as a punishment). On the contrary, the school staff seems to have taken this evidence very seriously, given careful thought as to how to respond and devised a method of dealing with the problem which (in my view) is probably at least as likely to be effective as any other kind of intervention. The school's offence, in the eyes of other sections of Danish society, is that (a) they did not follow the letter of the law and (b) they were afraid to confront these parents, or at any rate treated these children differently from other children, because of their cultural background, and because hitting at home was something that happened to 70% of the class. 'That 70% of children in a class are hit,' says the Children's Rights Organisation, 'does not make the problem any less serious for the individual child.'

With respect, the Children's Rights Organisation is talking simplistic nonsense. What is psychologically harmful about physical abuse is the message it gives to the child, and cultural context *does* make a difference to that message. I remember an observation made to me by a delightful Afrikaner student of mine who had grown up in a rural community in South Africa where it was normal for fathers to beat their children. He said he knew as a child that this was just what everyone's father did, and even when his father beat him he knew that his father loved him and that his father genuinely believed he was doing the right thing by his son. That might not make the beating *hurt* any less, but as a psychological experience it made it very different from an abusive beating given for no reason but anger and hate, even if the latter was physically no more painful and no more severe.

This is not to say that the authorities in Denmark are not perfectly entitled to insist that immigrant communities abide by Danish cultural norms and Danish law – not at all! – but the school did not dispute this. What the school did do was to try and find a way of trying to promote Danish cultural norms and Danish law in a way *that might actually work*, rather than respond in a rigid way that, in the judgement of school staff, would not achieve the objective of changing attitudes to violence in those communities, but would simply humiliate and alienate the parents and discourage the students from being honest with their teachers in future. This strikes me as intelligent and entirely defensible in terms of the likely outcomes of intervention. No method of intervention will be 100% effective at preventing the hitting of children, but I do not think there is a particularly strong case for believing that investigation of each family by local social care agencies would necessarily be any more effective.

But this still leaves us with a difficult question. Even if the school's actions could be justified in terms of likely outcomes, and in terms of showing appropriate respect to these children and their parents (and on both counts I think they could), could they be justified in terms of the teachers' obligations to the society that employs them? Or were these teachers behaving like those maverick detectives in American police movies who ignore the law and the rights of suspects on the basis that they know instinctively who the bad guys are and they know the only way to really stop them? Here we are up against some of the most difficult questions that face those of us who have to make ethical decisions not as private individuals but as representatives of organisations and servants of society as a whole.

It seems to me that behaving like a robot cannot be seen as a satisfactory ethical stance. The Nuremberg trials made clear that we cannot exonerate ourselves from personal moral responsibility simply by doing exactly what we are told. So the staff of this school showed moral courage by not just passing the problem on to the appropriate authorities and washing their hands of it. But nevertheless it would be a dangerous situation if professionals felt they could routinely ignore rules and procedures they did not personally agree with. Being a robot is not morally acceptable, but nor is being an unaccountable maverick (a 'loose cannon' as the English expression goes).

I think the most productive way forward would be for school staff to have talked to the appropriate authorities and tried to secure their agreement and cooperation in the approach they wanted to take. That way they would be contributing to thinking across society as a whole as to how to deal with these matters, rather than simply splitting themselves off from the rest of society and doing their own thing.

Easy for me to say, though, and harder in real-life situations when time is limited and where the scope for negotiation is not necessarily all that great. Sometimes the choice does seem to be between being a robot and being a maverick, and there does not seem to be much middle ground.

Chris Beckett is a Senior Lecturer in Social Work at the University of East Anglia, Norwich, England. He is the author of books on child protection and social work ethics. He dislikes corporal punishment and did not use it himself as a parent.

Questions for discussion about Case 5.4

1   Do you think the school was right to take the approach it did to tackling the issue of parents physically punishing their children?

2   The approach taken by the school could be regarded as 'culturally sensitive' practice, taking into account the fact that many of the families concerned were immigrants and refugees from Middle Eastern countries. What do you think is meant by 'culturally sensitive' practice, and how do you think it can be achieved, whilst also taking into account children's rights to non-violence, as recognised in Western countries?

3   Do you believe the Danish law forbidding physical punishment of children is a good law? What are the laws and regulations about physical punishment of children in your own country?

6 Working with policy and politics

Introduction

DEREK CLIFFORD

This chapter comprises case examples that deal with ethical problems that arise partly or wholly from policies, politics, laws and social and cultural structures that affect the lives of both social workers and service users. However individual and personal a problem might be, there is always a framework of policy, law and politics reflective of broad social divisions and differences of culture within which professional practitioners are permitted and/or required to intervene. These changing frameworks demand or facilitate certain types of intervention and discourage or disallow others. What may appear to be a very personal problem needing professional social intervention will always also be the outcome of multiple social, cultural and economic factors, and will be directly or indirectly influenced by the political or policy decisions of governments and organisations. This raises a number of questions:

- Once a social work case is understood within a broader context, how much are the ethical issues transformed?
- When a case is more directly influenced by policy, structural and cultural factors or political decisions, how can and how should social workers' ethical behaviour take this into account?
- How far should the ethics of the social professions focus on the

narrower horizons of interpersonal relationships, ignoring their embeddedness within wider social systems?

The political context of social work

Understanding the context within which social work currently operates requires some understanding of rapidly changing forces in modern societies. Many of these are at national and international levels, the most significant being the apparent triumph of global capitalism and the impact this has had on welfare provision across the world. As Schutte (2007: 172) comments:

> policies that appear to be only national in scope are in fact transnational, such as the increasing privatisation of formerly publicly funded education, health services and care giving services . . . [and the consequent] exploitive effects of global capitalism on the lives of Third World women.

The concentration of wealth and power in fewer hands entails the devolving of the impact of cyclical and other financial crises on those least able to resist it – both within and outside Western nations. This means that social professionals are increasingly required to intervene in ways predetermined by political and policy decisions, to shore up the political and economic system, providing minimal frameworks of support and control for allegedly dysfunctional and marginalised individuals and groups. A closely related factor is the hierarchical organisation of both public and private bodies: the model of business management has been widely incorporated into agencies in which social professionals work. One of the results of this development is that the wider picture is mediated through tightly controlled circumstances, undermining professionals' autonomous judgement and ability to relate to service users, but requiring detailed accountability procedures to ensure the efficient and profitable functioning of the organisation (Green 2009).

The traditional framing of social and community work values in many countries includes the recognition that individual, family and community problems cannot be understood only in terms of individual or local behaviours and simply be 'blamed' on them. The relationship between the individual and the surrounding environment has been one of continuing debate, and the rise of transnational corporations on the one hand and the green movement and the associated problems of global warming on the other, has given an added impetus to theories of social intervention that contextualise all practice within the framework of wider natural and social systems. However, the impact of social systems on individuals and communities has many antecedents, from Marx's emphasis on economic structures and Durkheim's insistence on the importance of cultural wholes, through to the social, informational and biological imperatives of 'scientific' systems theories.

By contrast, contemporary post-structuralist theories do not regard language as a transparent medium that connects one directly with a 'truth' or 'reality' and tend to question all these social and political explanations emphasising instead the fluidity and fragmentation of meanings. Yet the importance of wider factors can hardly be ignored. Within Western social work, as well as in wider circles, the use of systems and ecological theories remains high (Payne 1997: 137–156) and the political importance of systemic global interactions (such as financial crises and economic recession) and their impact on individual and community lives can hardly be overestimated, simultaneously raising issues of both respect and social justice, and social connection and responsibility (Gould 2009).

One of the demands of globalised capital is that individuals and organisations should be responsible for themselves in response to market demands for labour and in relation to the law, with the implication that individuals should be prepared to travel to wherever employment is on offer, and be prepared to pay for or accept whatever level of services the market will support. At the level of national states this can mean family and community disruption, when industries decline or global corporations relocate their investments to maximise their interests. A cross-cutting factor is the sociocultural variability manifested in social movements associated with groups often disproportionately at the receiving end. The fortunes of women, ethnic and religious groups, the physically and mentally disabled, gays and lesbians, young and old all variably interact with each other and with economic factors relating to poverty and social class in specific local circumstances conditioned by national and international forces (Martinez 2009). In addition, the occurrence of natural and human-made disasters and gross international inequalities of wealth encourage people to migrate to where they perceive safety and economic opportunity will be better, whilst the more vulnerable are left behind. Most modern states have to deal with internal social problems interconnected with demands arising from global poverty, insecurity and immigration, and the activities of global corporations, resulting in political and legal consequences for the social professions. Western countries face lower quality social welfare for vulnerable groups. Poorer countries are faced with the other end of this structurally determined inequality – the deprivation and often extreme poverty that arises from the ability of global corporations to exploit their low-waged and poorly organised workers, including women and children, sometimes referred to as 're-colonisation' (Schutte 2007: 165), and also the loss of qualified workers to more developed economies.

Implications for professional ethics

Ethical conceptions of the role of social professionals in mediating between the individual and wider society have included a variety of possibilities. It could be argued that a utilitarian concern with maximising benefits should guide policy and practice at institutional and personal levels, and that this underlies governments' concerns with 'good outcomes' (Banks 2004: 176). Managerialist trends in many contemporary states have pointed in this direction, led by powerful liberalising forces in Western economies, and additionally justified by moral and political arguments based on the rights of the possessive entrepreneurial individual and the minimal state (Nozick 1974). Classic utilitarianism is reflected in demands for achieving empirically researched best outcomes and targets, with accompanying inspection regimes and ethical compliance on the part of professionals. However, it has been a long-standing objection that values cannot be reduced to technical market efficiency, or simple moral rules alone, especially ones that reflect particular Western cultural and economic values. Case 6.3 (from Finland) illustrates the impact of global economic liberalism on the care of an older woman. How can carers – professional and 'voluntary' – manage to work ethically with policies designed to maximise organisational and financial outcomes at the cost of the dignity and welfare of individuals, especially older individuals who have worked all their lives, paying taxes, with an understanding that this would ensure care for them in their old age?

The human rights and equal opportunities values of liberal social and community workers are often set in contrast with the narrower utilitarian demands of the economy, and owe much to the arguments about justice put forward in the 1970s by John Rawls (1973) and also to the ethical demand for rational human dialogue proposed by Jürgen Habermas (1984), both drawing on Kantian ethics that contribute to a concern for liberty and social justice for individuals – but taking into account the social, economic and political context. They seek to argue for social and economic arrangements that will favour both the development of societies as a whole and the individuals within them. However, they also have their critics, who suggest they represent Western and male ideas that ignore the global position of exploited female workers. Feminist political philosophy and ethics (Held 2007; Young 1990) draw attention to the global as well as local interactions between a range of social divisions including gender, class, 'race', disability, sexuality and age, and challenge the implications of these forms of oppression for democratic socialist and feminist values, as well as professional social practice, (e.g., Tronto 2010), emphasising both care and power differentials. Young's (1990) work urges upon the reader the importance of placing the actions of professionals within the wider social context, and is itself explicitly developed from ideas drawn from social movements of the late twentieth century.

On the other hand the rediscovery of ancient ideas about virtue theory by contemporary moral philosophers and postmodernists has placed a focus on the character of the moral actor, and the importance of qualities such as courage in the face of systemic and structural obstacles (Banks and Gallagher 2009). Case 6.4 raises difficult questions about how professionals should try to realise justice and welfare for an abused young woman in Palestine, where child protection law and policy are at a developmental stage; where the relevant community values have a massive influence over what can and should be done; and where there is an overarching political situation of unresolved conflict. How far can and should professionals act with integrity and courage in relation to their own values of protecting vulnerable young women, and what compromises might be regarded as justifiable in the light of both community values and political constraints? The implications for practice of an understanding of the wider context within which social professionals work would not necessarily be the same if different perspectives are taken on social justice, social difference and care.

Taking account of the bigger picture

The wider frameworks within which social professionals have to make difficult ethical decisions reconfigure the understanding that might be brought to bear on any proposed intervention at different levels. Being a member of a particular society leaves a professional *more or less* committed to the values and laws of that society, depending on how far they identify with and approve of the moral value of the political and social arrangements. If local values are prioritised over the beliefs of other societies, then this *may* raise questions about the ethical justification for aid to wider humanity, rather than to the existing members of a particular state, and how individuals and societies should discharge their responsibilities to others, including the global poor (see Pogge 2006). In Western societies the usual assumption is that if a law has been properly enacted, by a governing political party that has some kind of electoral mandate from voters in a free election, society can legitimately expect that those laws and the local values they express should be obeyed – or individuals will face the legal consequences. Professionals cannot ethically or prudentially afford to ignore such considerations – even in countries where there is little evidence of shared values, legitimacy or probity in government or sympathy for wider humanity. How far should professionals accommodate their actions towards central and local powers that may not be sympathetic to professional values, and whose representatives may 'legitimately' or 'illegitimately' make questionable demands? This ethical dilemma is very apparent in Case 6.2, where professionals in Pakistan have to make difficult judgements about how far they can ethically compromise their position before deciding to withdraw from a situation, knowing that service users may suffer as a consequence.

Additionally, professionals cannot ignore the possibility that legitimately processed laws and policies may be ethically unacceptable, expressing, for instance, the racism and xenophobia that arises in many countries where incomers are treated at best as second-class providers of labour. However, societies are not monolithic and the fact that people hold a variety of religious, social and moral values can give rise to critical reflection on the moral worth of policies and laws. In addition, societies are ever more interrelated with other societies in an age of globalised communication. Professionals thus need to consider how ethical a proposed action might be to a *number* of possible audiences that can claim to have a stake in the proposed action – both within their own societies at the local level of organisation and community, and at the interconnected wider national and transnational levels, both of which now impinge increasingly closely on local decision-making. The stake that service users and carers and their organisations have in the proposed action is a vital set of claims that has to be contextualised against that background.

The challenge for social professionals

In the cases included in this chapter we see professionals struggling to reflect upon the ethical issues that arise in their work and to take actions that appear to answer some of their ethical concerns. A common feature is how they understand the situation they are in – from a very wide angle that includes their own social location, thoroughly examining the wider picture. They realise that their ethical reflections and subsequent actions inevitably take on a 'political' element insofar as they are forced to choose to pursue a course of action that others would contest. This may involve deliberate opposition to and subversion of agency policies and/or government policy and law, as in Case 6.1 about working with refugees in Australia. Here the social worker was clear that a policy legally enacted by the government and politically supported was ethically unacceptable and needed to be opposed. How can professionals ethically oppose policies and statutes whilst working for an agency that is charged with carrying them out? How far can professionals risk their own position and concern themselves with values and policy rather than focus on the immediate needs of service users? Sometimes there may be little that can or should be done immediately to affect a situation that is highly structured by hierarchical agencies and dictatorial governments (both Western and non-Western). However, such situations should still be thought through on the basis of an awareness of what those structures are, and how this might suggest an agenda and a strategy for the future, if the needs of vulnerable people are not being met.

What a professional considers to be unjust or oppressive treatment of either individuals or groups is a matter that many social movements in the twentieth century began to bring to public awareness – raising the appreciation of the needs of differing social groups. The lack of shared values between and within societies, stemming from the experience of different cultures, politics and religions means that social professionals have an impossible task – yet one that cannot be refused. To think ethically about the 'wider picture' is to think ethically and politically about themselves and the world in which they live. The cases in this chapter provide evidence that although a difficult task, it can be done, it has to be done, and it is worth doing.

References

Banks, S. (2004) *Ethics Accountability and the Social Professions*, Basingstoke, UK: Palgrave Macmillan.

Banks, S. and Gallagher, A. (2009) *Ethics in Professional Life: Virtues for Health and Social Care*, Basingstoke, UK: Palgrave Macmillan.

Gould, C. C. (2009) 'Varieties of global responsibility: social connection, human rights and transnational solidarity', in A. Ferguson and N. Mechthild (eds) *Dancing with Iris: The Philosophy of Iris Marion Young*, Oxford: Oxford University Press.

Green, J. (2009) 'The deformation of professional formation: managerial targets and the undermining of professional judgement', *Ethics and Social Welfare*, 3(2): 115–130.

Habermas, J. (1984) *Theory of Communicative Action, Volume 1: Reason and the Rationalisation of Society*, translated by T. McCarthy, London: Heinemann.

Held, V. (2007) *The Ethics of Care: Personal, Political and Global*, Oxford: Oxford University Press.

Martinez, M. (2009) 'On immigration politics in the context of European societies and the structural inequality model', in A. Ferguson and N.

Mechthild (eds) *Dancing with Iris: The Philosophy of Iris Marion Young*, Oxford: Oxford University Press.

Nozick, R. (1974) *Anarchy, State and Utopia*, Oxford: Blackwell.

Payne, M. (1997) *Modern Social Work Theory*, 2nd edition, Basingstoke: Macmillan.

Pogge, T. (2006) 'Migration and poverty', in R. E. Goodin and P. Petit (eds) *Contemporary Political Philosophy*, Oxford: Blackwell.

Rawls, J. (1973) *A Theory of Justice*, Oxford: Oxford University Press.

Schutte, O. (2007) 'Postcolonial feminisms: genealogies and recent directions', in L. Alcoff and E. Kittay (eds) *The Blackwell Guide to Feminist Philosophy*, Oxford: Blackwell.

Tronto, J. (2010) 'Creating caring institutions: politics, plurality, and purpose', *Ethics and Social Welfare*, 4(2): 158–171.

Young, I. M. (1990) *Justice and the Politics of Difference*, Princeton, NJ: Princeton University Press.

Case study 6.1

Case 6.1   Challenging pernicious policies: working with refugees in Australia

Introduction

This case is about the concerns of a social work practitioner in stretching the boundaries of her everyday work in a refugee settlement agency in Australia. The context of the case is the mandatory detention of asylum seekers in Australia and their release into the community, which from 1999 to 2008 resulted in the granting of restrictive temporary visa status only. This case is compiled by an academic convenor of the People's Inquiry into Detention[1] based on a conversation with a social work service provider who gave an account of how she had struggled to resolve the following issues:

1   how to find a way to meet the needs of asylum seekers released from immigration detention who are not entitled to services; and
2   whether to speak publicly about damaging policies and practices when a culture of organisational silence pervades.

[1] The findings of the People's Inquiry into Detention are documented in Briskman, L., Latham, S. and Goddard, C. (2008) *Human Rights Overboard: Seeking Asylum in Australia*, Melbourne: Scribe. The book won the 2008 Australian Human Rights Commission award for literature (non-fiction).

The case

Jennifer is an experienced social worker employed in a refugee settlement agency funded by the government. In accordance with the funding contract, the service she provides is to assist with the settlement of refugees who arrive in Australia through the United Nations High Commissioner for Refugees processes, usually after spending years in overseas refugee camps. Her NGO receives the bulk of its funding from government. The organisation employs a mix of social work and non-social work staff. One of Jennifer's roles is the training of volunteers to assist with the work.

In 2005, Jennifer was confronted with some dilemmas. She became increasingly concerned about the policies of the Australian government towards asylum seekers, who arrived by boat and were mandatorily detained in immigration centres where they sometimes languished for many years. When these people were eventually recognised as refugees they were released on Temporary Protection Visas (TPVs) with few rights and were prohibited from access to settlement services.

Many people on TPVs turned up at Jennifer's organisation only to be told they were not eligible for assistance. Their only recourse was to approach one of a small number of charitable groups that had sprung up in an endeavour to fill the gap. These organisations were under-resourced, funded by small donations and had lengthy waiting lists. The volunteers they had gathered to assist required training and support, particularly as they were often dealing with traumatised people.

Jennifer decided to take a number of courses of action. Firstly, she joined a refugee advocacy group to assist people on TPVs in her spare time, drawing on the knowledge derived from her work. This included training volunteers. She did not advise her employer of this involvement. Secondly, she wrote a confidential submission to the People's Inquiry into Detention about her experiences with people who were denied services. The People's Inquiry had been established by a group of academic social workers (Australian Council of Heads of Schools of Social Work) in order to receive testimonies about immigration detention so that the policies and practices were documented and exposed.

Jennifer grappled with some ethical questions. The Australian Association of Social Workers (AASW) Code of Ethics (1999)[2] espouses a broad commitment to social justice and calls on social workers to act

2 Australian Association of Social Workers (1999, 2nd edition 2002) *AASW Code of Ethics*, Kingston, ACT: AASW. The 1999 version (2nd edition 2002) was in operation at the time. The code was revised in 2010. Both versions can be found at www.aasw.asn.au/publications/ethics-and-standards

to change social structures that preserve inequalities and injustice. The code also specifies that social workers should strive to carry out the aims and objectives of their employing bodies while challenging and working to improve policies and practices.

Jennifer did not feel she could challenge or subvert the workplace policies as the organisation was dependent on government funding. Although she had not signed a confidentiality agreement, there was a tacit rule that she should not speak out about unjust policies as the programme funding may be put in jeopardy, which would then put another group of clients at risk. Instead she subverted the system by offering advice to refugees, advocates and volunteers based on her professional knowledge and experience, but outside the organisational realm.

Jennifer anguished about speaking out to the People's Inquiry. Although the Inquiry was run by social workers, she realised that the academics had a greater degree of freedom and less organisational constraints in their advocacy. After speaking to organisers of the People's Inquiry she decided to submit a confidential statement about the problems with lack of service provision and the cruel bar on family reunion which affected people on TPVs. She knew that the AASW was supportive of the Inquiry and hoped that if she was 'caught out' she would have the backing of the profession. She did not seek advice on this as she became determined to act and did not want any barriers put in her way.

When Jennifer spoke about how she was troubled about what to do, she explained how she reached her decision. She said she gave priority to her belief that social workers had a professional and moral obligation to ensure that all people had access to services. She also stressed that the wider community needed to be informed of the existing injustices. In deciding to take action, she came to the view that acting to restore justice overrode obligations to her employing organisation.

Even though the People's Inquiry was held under the auspices of a social work organisation, only a handful of social workers spoke out. As few social workers were employed within immigration detention facilities they had not had the same level of direct contact with asylum seekers as had groups such as nurses, psychiatrists and psychologists. There was also little organised activity among social work practitioners and it would have been difficult for social workers to act alone in making a stance. As Jennifer was able directly to witness the suffering arising post-detention, she had the knowledge to act in ways she believed were appropriate and also to speak out about the suffering. As she was an experienced social worker, she had confidence in her actions.

Commentary 1

SEMA BUZ AND EMRAH AKBAŞ

This case exemplifies the general policy trend in many countries in relation to refugees. In most European countries, for instance, the general trend is to exclude refugees from mainstream society, and, if possible, to not receive any refugees at all, or to force them to return by means of rigid policies that restrict access to basic social welfare services.

At the time when this case is set (2005), asylum seekers arriving in Australia stay in immigration centres, often for several years, and when they gain refugee status they receive Temporary Protection Visas (TPVs). However, this does not entitle them to have their basic needs met. This is in total opposition to the principle of social justice, since the refugees encounter many inequalities, injustice and exclusion. What refugees are exposed to in this case highlights the fact that the Australian government violates international standards for refugee protection.

As to Jennifer's attitude and behaviour, she complains about the results of the unjust policies regarding refugees because she has trouble in reaching the resources for meeting the basic needs of the refugees. And she takes some actions to overcome this. As a social justice value, she tries to work in solidarity with colleagues in order to create equal access to resources. However, her endeavour for solidarity does not seem to include the refugees, but only colleagues and service providers. The account given here does not depict a participatory practice in which service users are involved as agents.

In struggling against the unjust policies and practices, what Jennifer does is only to reach a group of advocates composed of academic social workers, but she keeps silent within the agency. Jennifer experiences a dilemma within the agency in relation to speaking out about the unjust policies, but her opposition directly focuses on the agency's position, not on the general refugee policies of the government. As a political agent the social worker should also be prepared to take action against unjust policies – sometimes leading social action initiatives composed of the general public and service users. However, in this case what Jennifer does is restricted to joining two action groups, which does not appear to result in immediately effective results. Social action is an indispensable dimension of social work practice since social workers have an ethical responsibility to society. In struggling against unjust policies, a social worker is supposed to take notice of her managers, decision-making mechanisms, politicians and the general public.

Jennifer joins the group of social work academics, but in this account no mention is made of being in solidarity with colleagues in the professional associations. Professional associations are perhaps the main actors for challenging government policies, and could be contacted as part of Jennifer's ethical responsibility towards the profession itself. She could also seek other ways of working in solidarity, for instance she could communicate at the international and global level with the International Federation of Social Workers.

To conclude, we have several suggestions to overcome the dilemmas Jennifer experienced. First, she should engage in a more politically-oriented action by applying to her national association of social workers in order to challenge the unjust policies in a national arena, representing the voice of all the social workers in the country. It is possible to create an international and global platform or network only after achieving a national-level awareness and endeavour. Second, she should be well aware of the fact that the service users themselves are both the agents of their lives and they also must be political actors fighting against what they suffer. So she should seek ways to develop participatory social action. Third, although she is aware of and uncomfortable about the organisational silence, as an ethical responsibility she should make efforts to challenge, or at least make representations to, her managers within the NGO.

Finally, at the heart of this problem lies the fact that what Jennifer is exposed to is not her own dilemma, but the dilemma of the profession itself witnessing the transformation of the system of delivery of social services in a way that is in opposition to the ethical principles of the profession itself. So it is important to be aware of a bigger picture, focusing more on the structures determining the single acts. What Jennifer is supposed to do as a social worker is to notice her ethical responsibility to the profession. Thus, any act in which she is involved must also include consideration of the structures shaping the profession itself.

Sema Buz Ph.D. is Associate Professor in the Department of Social Work, Faculty of Economics and Administrative Sciences, Hacettepe University, Turkey.

Emrah Akbaş Ph.D. is Lecturer in the Department of Social Work, Faculty of Economics and Administrative Sciences, Hacettepe University, Turkey.

Commentary 2

LINDA HARMS SMITH

This case relates to the conflict around constraint in adequate service provision through the enforcement of national and organisational policies. It seems that the organisation and the social worker in this case have similar aims, that is, providing appropriate services to refugees. It is in the interpretation of what is necessary and possible that they differ, primarily due to the dictates and authority of the government funding institution. Being limited by the prevailing status quo versus challenging and resisting it becomes an ethical struggle.

The social worker seems morally courageous in her willingness to subvert the system and pursue what she believes is right. However, answering various questions and pursuing further strategies may allow for even stronger position-taking, challenge the tacit rule of silence imposed by the organisation and in the longer term achieve greater levels of social justice.

Key ethical issues

The struggle around pursuing actions which address problems of injustice, discrimination and inequality, while at the same time meeting needs only partially in order to adhere to policy and so leaving the status quo unchallenged, is perennial.

It may be argued that social work as a profession arose from the consequences of an unjust world economic order, acting as a palliative for and servant to these structural dynamics. And so social work often finds itself in a position of acquiescence and complicity with ongoing oppression and maintenance of the status quo.

When considering the case description, the following further ethical issues emerge:

- Whether to speak out ('truth-telling' or the 'parrhesiastic' act) about socially unjust and damaging policies versus adhering to a tacit rule about organisational silence.
- Exercising status quo maintenance and social control functions versus taking a stand for social justice and social change through advocacy and collectivist approaches.
- Challenging hegemonic discourse versus acquiescence to taken-for-granted power dynamics of the funding and recipient organisation.

- Focus of efforts on human potential, agency and personal responsibility versus focus on the political and structural.
- Maintaining professional integrity as a morally active practitioner versus acting for organisational interests and employer/employee contractual requirements.
- Adhering to organisational policies and maintaining the status quo versus challenging policy and contributing to social change.

Universal/general questions

This social worker's struggle is a universal one. Being constrained by dictates of funding and policy, in the face of unjust, damaging policies and laws, is the nature of the conflicted and discomforted position of the social worker. Discrimination against and violation of refugees' rights is an example of any social injustice and human rights violation, temporally or geographically – whether the context is past South African apartheid policy or current European austerity measures. In the South African context, working as a social worker during apartheid with its gross human rights violations posed daily ethical dilemmas around resisting the status quo and subverting and challenging injustice. As in this case, vigilance, truth-telling and advocacy about structural oppressions pose a measure of risks of professional alienation, loss of employment or even consequences of coming into conflict with the law.

It is not only within oppressive societies that socio-economic injustice, inequality and damaging laws and policies prevail. These are also evident in so-called free and affluent societies. Hegemonic structural arrangements and internalisation of oppressive social relations occur even in transformed societies. Globally, prevailing neo-liberal capitalist ideologies create high levels of inequality, discriminate against people and violate human rights. Social workers face consequences and risks as a result of their commitments to social change and working towards a better world.

Actions taken by the social worker

Conscientisation around injustice She joined a refugee advocacy group in her spare time . . . the wider community needed to be informed of the existing injustices.

- What was her obligation to management around creating awareness about these injustices and confronting and deconstructing ideological persuasions? Would her lengthy experience as a social worker not contribute to greater respect for her views? Would this advice have been useful within the organisational framework? What conscientisation efforts within the organisation may have shifted positions on these issues?

Respecting the tacit rule of silence   There was a tacit rule that she should not speak out about unjust policies.

- Was there really an obligation to the organisation to remain silent and leave injustice unchallenged? Did this 'tacit rule' really need to be accepted given that there was no contractual obligation? Was this a case of a lack of assertive behaviour on the social worker's part?

Avoiding funding being placed in jeopardy   The programme funding would be put in jeopardy if anyone spoke out about unjust policies.

- Was the assumption that the programme funding would be in jeopardy correct? Might there have been other sources of funding? Would the shift in unjust policies through activism and conscientisation benefit service users in the long term?

Subversion of the system   She subverted the system by offering advice to refugees, advocates and volunteers outside the organisational realm.

- Was the advice that she was able to offer refugees, advocates and volunteers really subversive? How would the organisation and its service users have benefited from similar input? What restoration of justice would have been possible in the organisational context?

Advocacy efforts   There was little organised activity among social work practitioners and it would have been difficult to act alone. A confidential submission to the People's Inquiry into Detention was written.

- What collective approaches might have been utilised? What shifts in unjust policies might political activism have achieved? What were the positions of management regarding these issues? Might the organisation have been able to prepare a confidential submission to the People's Inquiry? What, if any, formal avenues were available for policy advocacy? How might the service user group be included in advocacy efforts?

Conclusion

Social work is political. The dialectical tension between focusing on human agency and focusing on structural problems causes ethical struggles. These become more complicated when organisational and statutory policies are part of what is unjust and damaging. When confronted with clear and unambiguous social injustice it may be easier to take a stand and participate in social action and advocacy efforts. However, when hegemonic orders prevail and global economic and social injustice is the order of the day it is harder to challenge these inequalities and oppressions. If social workers want to pursue social justice and equality they will have to embrace their discomforted and conflicted positions and engage in truth-telling, advocacy, collective action and political interventions.

Linda Harms Smith is Lecturer in Social Work at the University of Witwatersrand, South Africa.

Questions for discussion about Case 6.1

1   When faced with situations of systematic injustice as described in this case, what factors should a social worker take into account in deciding what action to take?
2   Jennifer took two courses of action: joining a refuge advocacy group outside work; and making a confidential submission to the People's Inquiry. Neither of these involved her directly challenging her employer or government policies, but clearly both required courage and commitment. What other courses of action might be open to social workers in similar situations? How would you justify them ethically?
3   If social workers are to take responsibility to report injustice and to 'blow the whistle' on bad, inhumane and degrading practice, what support do they need?

Case 6.2 Maintaining organisational integrity in an area of conflict: a women's NGO in Pakistan

Introduction

This case is about a non-governmental organisation (NGO) working with women and children in the Federally Administered Tribal Areas of Pakistan. This area is poorly developed, and women are severely restricted in what they can do. They are not, for example, allowed by their male relatives to see male medical staff or meet women outside their family other than for approved activities such as collecting water. An estimated three per cent of women can read, the rates for child and mother mortality are among the highest in the world and poverty is grinding, with smuggling and drug-running being among the most lucrative activities. In addition to these problems the area is very unsafe. Households are more likely to own Kalashnikov rifles than to have access to clean water. The Taliban dominate much of the area and exert their authority by force.

The case

A women's and children's NGO, *Khwendo Kor*, has set itself the task of providing health, education and advocacy services to women and children in the Federally Administered Tribal Areas (FATA) and Khyber Pakhtunkhwa of Pakistan. The NGO is locally run and was established in the early 1990s by a woman who is herself from FATA and remains the Chief Executive. Starting from a staff of four, Khwendo Kor now employs more than 300 staff, runs over 200 schools for girls, has trained over 1,000 traditional birth attendants, runs micro-credit schemes and female adult literacy classes and helps women obtain identity cards and vote in elections. It receives funding primarily from overseas donors.

The backdrop to these achievements makes them all the more remarkable given that FATA is very poorly developed, is among the most conservative areas in the world and is dominated by the Taliban. Traditionally, the Taliban do not approve of female education and staff from the NGO are at risk of being shot or kidnapped, and their offices have been bombed. Their ability to work in the area at all depends on negotiations with whoever has power in the particular villages they target. The ability to conciliate those in power is thus crucial to their ability to work in the area at all and often to the safety of their staff. If this initial negotiation is successful, Khwendo Kor then has to approach the men in the village and only through them can they eventually work with the women. The NGO involves *maliks* (headmen) in its activities at all stages of its interventions. However, this is not easy. The maliks usually ask for personal favours such as jobs, monetary incentives, and the upper hand in decision-making. The following two examples illustrate some of the issues for Khwendo Kor.

1   In a village in *Khyber agency*, the acting malik agreed to support a girls' school and one of his female relatives was appointed as a teacher. However, later he insisted that his brother be employed as the Khwendo Kor's field supervisor and asked for a rise in the salary of the female teacher beyond the NGO rules. He avoided the collective community meetings and insisted on his demands. Although the other members agreed to have a second teacher from outside the village, the malik said he would not be able to take responsibility for her security. At this point the Programme Director insisted that Khwendo Kor could not go beyond certain limits in compromising its principles, and eventually the school had to be shifted to a nearby village. The reasons for the decision were that the acting malik had showed himself to be too powerful to allow the village community itself to make collective decisions with regard to education. In such situations the withdrawal of support from one person (the malik) could jeopardise the whole enterprise and female education could collapse. Although fewer students were enrolled in the new school (at least initially) and only a handful of girls from the original school were allowed by their families to attend, the involvement from the 'new' village through the establishment of a men's education committee and a women's education committee was far greater, thus putting it onto a much firmer footing. Khwendo Kor learnt from this experience that it should not move ahead with its education plans without a broad base of effective support from the wider community, even if an individual in a highly influential position is supportive and the early soundings look positive. It also learnt the importance of Khwendo Kor senior staff being aware of interactions between influential villagers and more junior staff. For example, it was the malik's attitude to the latter that first started the alarm bells ringing about the insecurity of the situation; this had not been apparent in the dealings of senior staff with him.

Although Khwendo Kor itself decided to withdraw from the school, it took the decision to leave the teachers behind and negotiate for the government to provide some input into its continuation.

2 Similarly, in *FR Bannu* a malik allowed the traditional training of birth attendants to take place on condition that it was only for his wife and a few close female relatives. This malik was influential outside his village as well and the NGO needed his blessing to work in the area. Members of Khwendo Kor staff do not usually provide the training for fewer than 10–12 women, but they decided to proceed because the area was a stronghold of the Taliban and any invitation to make inroads was to be welcomed. Therefore the NGO agreed to provide the traditional birth attendants' training to only three women. This then resulted in the wife of the malik getting paid employment in a government Basic Health Unit in his village. However, after achieving his personal objective, this malik became disinterested in the NGO and did not support them against the Taliban. Soon after the training was delivered the security situation in the area deteriorated. Khwendo Kor had to close their local office and withdraw their staff. However, Khwendo Kor continues to believe that their approach was sound. The fact that the wife went on to become employed by the government as a result of receiving the training will, they believe, have some benefits. She will act as a role model for other local women insofar as she received training from an 'outside' women's NGO and is now employed outside the home – and this was with the support of the wider village community. The malik's increased income (the wife's salary will go directly to him) is likely to provide him with an incentive to support women's development in the future, perhaps when the security situation eases and Khwendo Kor is able to reopen their office.

The dilemmas faced by Khwendo Kor are often to do with knowing when their approach is acceptably pragmatic and when it has tipped over into risking the compromise of their values. There are times when the delivery of a service can appear to be effective (or hold the potential to be) but can jeopardise the safety of staff, collude with activities which might be regarded as corrupt, undermine its sustainability or otherwise compromise the values that the organisation purports to uphold.

Commentary 1

IAN SINCLAIR

I will explore what I see as the main dilemma for the NGO in this case, which was whether or not to go along with a practice that could be seen as corrupt.

If the NGO did as the maliks wanted it would arguably condone corruption. It might also face practical consequences. Western donors who might hear what happened might be less willing to provide funding. Other maliks might feel that similar exceptions should be made for them. The NGO might find that it had to take on inefficient or lazy staff and provide training for groups when it was not economic to do so. Both the integrity and the cost effectiveness of the programme might be threatened.

By contrast a refusal to go along with those who had power locally could also have consequences. The NGO operates in the Federally Administered Tribal Areas (FATA) and focuses its work on women and children. This is dangerous work. The area is fought over by the Pakistan Army and the Taliban who distrust NGOs, particularly those promoting female education. The NGO's offices have been bombed, some staff have been kidnapped and others wounded in shootings; death threats are common. It is only through its ability to work with those with local power, and through them to reach the people in the villages, that the NGO is able to survive, get the facilities it needs for its schools and other work, and be warned when it is dangerous to be about. And in this case it risked alienating local men with power and thus jeopardising the work it wanted to do.

There is a further consideration. The organisation's moral purpose gives meaning and coherence to its work, enables it to maintain financial integrity despite the low wages it has to pay its staff, and maintains its morale. An overly pragmatic stance risks giving a mixed message to staff about what is and is not acceptable. Thus, whatever stance the NGO takes on these issues it is important that it is clear and coherent.

What ethical principles might enable the NGO to thread its way through these dilemmas? I would suggest three, which are outlined below.

First, its overriding 'mission' must be feasible and focused. Its job is to better the lot of the women and children in its area. It cannot afford to take on other battles unless they are both winnable and clearly relevant to its mission. The battle against corruption is not its central concern.

Second, this mission must be pursued 'honourably'. Thus, while the NGO has not made the battle against corruption its central focus, it has refused to pay bribes to officials who demanded them as a condition of providing further grants.

Third, the mission has to be pursued pragmatically and with due regard to local customs. In the Western world the *burqa* (veil) may be seen as a symbol of women's oppression. It is not so seen in FATA and staff from the NGO wear the burqa in those areas where this is demanded. Similarly, a Western agency might have no difficulty in paying a local man for use of a facility. In the context of FATA, the maliks risk their lives by supporting this NGO. Is it unreasonable for them to demand payment in the form of employing their relatives, if they can do the job?

These principles need to be balanced. So the need for pragmatism can conflict with the need for a clear moral stance, and the need for focus with that for an 'honourable' stance. This conflict of principles is just a matter of how life is. Philosophers seem to distinguish between ethical systems in terms of whether they emphasise the consequences of actions, the rules that should govern them, or their implications for the moral character of the agent. In the real world these considerations have to be put together. So in the analogous case of an organisation, it has to consider consequences, set itself rules and maintain a 'moral character'.

Viewed from this perspective the case shows the NGO in a good light. It kept its focus on its mission of serving the women and children in FATA. It acted pragmatically and in a culturally sensitive way, going along with problematic demands in the light of the need to achieve its wider aim. It was, however, conscious that this could be 'a slippery slope', which is illustrated by the example of the girls' school. When a threshold was crossed, the NGO felt that its work in that particular village was no longer viable and shifted its efforts to another.

Ian Sinclair is Emeritus Professor of Social Work, University of York, UK.

Commentary 2

GRACY FERNANDES

The first example: the school in Khyber agency

The political context

The events described in the functioning of this NGO in Pakistan, Khwendo Kor, highlight the fragile community and NGO situation, despite the apparent success of Khwendo Kor and its efforts for female education.

The political scenario is complex and displays the power struggle among the key players – the Programme Director of Khwendo Kor, the staff, the malik-headman and the Taliban personnel. The client system is the community, particularly the women. However, their voices and views do not surface openly, although it is mentioned that the involvement of the men's education committee and the women's education committee was far greater in shifting the school to a nearby village. The circumstances indicate that the power is wielded by a male, the malik, who uses his role to further the position of his family members in the NGO and holds the NGO to ransom in demanding a rise in the salary beyond the NGO rules. While the NGO negotiates logically and is brave in insisting on its administrative and functional principles by proposing alternatives, the NGO is at a loss without any assurance by the malik of the security of the second teacher from outside the village.

The lessons learnt by the NGO

In the context of the difficult political situation, the NGO has learnt important lessons, namely the role of the wider community. For the success of the education programme, the support of family and community strength is crucial. The NGO has also calculated that, even if it did its best to gain this community support, there are factors, such as the powerful political situation, that are beyond its control. Ultimately, the political situation is one of the major hurdles for any social and economic progress of the community.

The efforts made by the NGO to find an alternative solution demonstrate that in the current political situation the domination of powerful people affects the entire community – because the education plan is in the interest of the community women and girls. In the long run, if the entire community and the NGO persevere in their conviction and remain united in their search for the common good, they eventually will have a crucial role in being a counter power to be reckoned with. This also takes account of the interactions between influential villagers and the junior staff.

Ethical issues involved

This example underlines several implications for social work practice:

- It highlights aspects of religion, ideologies, traditional cultures and beliefs.

- It focuses on how these factors work either to mitigate conflict and search for resolution and reconciliation, or, in this case, encourage conflicts and destabilise the efforts of the NGO to strengthen the community base and women's and girls' welfare through education.
- Further, this conflicting situation demonstrates which section of the population is vulnerable and prone to be affected in situations of political instability.
- This case displays how, in the name of 'Islamic culture', the male dominating power leads to the subjugation of women and particularly of the younger women.

The key ethical dilemma facing the NGO is that of preserving its objectives, values and convictions, while confronting the threats of the Taliban dominated region and the power of influential individuals. It is commendable to note the negotiating skills of the NGO in proposing alternative interventions to safeguard the education of girls. Even though it does not meet with evident success, the NGO upholds its integrity. This incident exemplifies how in a given political situation where the Taliban is pervasive, the media can mobilise international social work support to strengthen local policy and service effectiveness in girls' education, especially with limited resources. Social workers can report to funding agencies on the progress of the outcomes of their interventions in their region. At the heart of this problem lies the persevering 'moral force' of the NGO, with risks to its personnel. There is no ready-made answer. As social workers we can try non-violent communication, reconciliation and aim for a proactive, collaborative and participatory approach to move ahead without any concluding solutions.

In times of violent political conflict, social workers cannot rigidly apply the international code of ethics. We need to assess the contextual and local situation and seek to influence strategic local policy towards social justice in terms of the feasibility of intervention, duty-based ethics and values of the NGOs. This situation underlines that these events are beyond the social work profession and ethics. Could the NGO seek collective support from national and international women's organisations and human rights groups? Are social workers ready to face personal and professional risks, even to their lives, in such situations?

The second example: training for birth attendants in FR Bannu

Struggle between the powerful and the powerless

This incident clearly illustrates how the malik uses his power to serve his own personal gains rather than the common good of the entire community. He also uses the 'Talibanised' political situation to further his position. In this situation, when the parties are unequal (the malik is powerful and the NGO is, seemingly, much less powerful), it is the NGO that runs the risk of compromising its greater goals and values for the collective good. This circumstance also shows that, sometimes, the only way of avoiding such compromise for an NGO faced with a powerful individual malik dictating and profiting at the cost of collective gains is to withdraw its service.

Ethical issues

The political situation is volatile and risky. As mentioned earlier the NGO compromises its values in allowing the powerful individual to take the upper hand in terms of reducing the number of women to be trained. This is a good example of the tussle between the powerful and the powerless. The powerful safeguard and assure the interests of their family members. The NGO is aware of the risks in maintaining its own convictions. There is also an element of fear should the NGO or other community members confront the malik.

This unpleasant incident illustrates the dilemmas in times of political crises, when the powerful dominate and instil fear, even at the risk of compromising value. This situation has similarities with the current political crises in Madagascar (where I work at present), where the ancestral culture is sacred and has to be respected at all costs. It is the elders and the powerful that dictate and make decisions that others have to follow, although they do not always agree. It is disrespectful to show dissent, especially if you are young, and you have to consent for fear of dire consequences. Those in power seek to ensure that their family members benefit from the services meant for all, as in the case of employment – safeguarding family interest or the 'red tape' (bureaucratic) model. Social work practitioners have an important role to play in empowering the community with knowledge, skills of communication and negotiation. In this case, the NGO is aware of the unjust and corrupt state of affairs, but is realistic and pragmatic. The staff accept the judgement of the NGO to compromise in the greater interest, despite the fact that they would like to uphold their convictions and values at a great risk to their personal lives and to the NGO.

A key issue that arises is the role of the individual social worker in dangerous and difficult situations like this. How far can the social worker take a stand that supports or goes against the decision of the local NGO in political conflict? There are other obvious questions in the context of the larger uncertainty and of how best to intervene in this complex political and social reality. To what extent are social workers ready to pay the price of holding on to their personal and professional values? Are they willing to risk their lives?

An analogous, if subtly different, set of dilemmas faces the NGO. We hear that the NGO offices have been bombed, and staff are at risk of being shot and kidnapped. In the face of such critical events, the NGO is in a 'no win situation', having to choose between compromising its effectiveness and mission to the local population while endangering its staff or appearing to go along with the ethically dubious position of powerful individuals.

The reality faced by Khwendo Kor is indicative of the personal, professional and ethical issues confronting the helping and humanitarian professions on the international scene today. Such incidents pose some critical reflections on personal and professional values, the nature of service intervention in times of violent political scenarios and the role of the international community in seeking resolution in such circumstances. When the local populations are the victims of military force and terrorism as in Pakistan, the major question then is: What is the role of NGOs, be they local, national or international? Is it time that the International Federation of Social Workers and the international organisations of social work offered help in some measures to protect the affected and vulnerable sections of society, especially women and children? And what recourse and mechanisms of assistance could be made available to NGOs and social work professionals?

Gracy Fernandes is a researcher, and is a member of the social work faculty and in charge of the Department of Programmes for Research and Continued Training at the Institut Supérieur de Travail Social, Antananarivo, Madagascar. She taught philosophy and ethics in the College of Social Work, Mumbai, and co-authored a book, *An Enquiry into Ethical Dilemmas in Social Work* (College of Social Work, Nirmala Niketan, 2006).

Questions for discussion about Case 6.2

1 Clearly this NGO has a set of ideals and ethical principles which influence its decisions about where and how to work. From the information in this case study, what do you think these might be?
2 Does the *end* (goal) of this NGO (women's and children's education and empowerment) justify the *means* used (acknowledging and working with the power of the maliks) to achieve this end?
3 Working for women's empowerment in an area of violent, political conflict with a strong tradition of male domination is a high-risk project. If you were the manager of such a project, how would you ensure adequate provision for the support and safety of staff and service users?

Case study 6.3

Case 6.3 The shrinking welfare state: caring for older people in Finland

Introduction

This case comes from eastern Finland and is written by a carer – the daughter of an older woman recently diagnosed with Alzheimer's disease. Finland has traditionally had a comprehensive system of welfare services provided by the national and local state, developed following the Second World War. However, public services are now being reformed and cut back in Finland. This has particularly profound consequences for older people in more remote rural areas, as this case illustrates.

The case

January 07 – Asking for help
I woke up at 4:30 a.m. when my mother, Maria, aged 75 years, telephoned me. She was in an exceptionally agitated state and blamed me for interfering in her banking business. It was hard to understand what she

was talking about. Something was missing or wrong. I was confused. My father had died only six months ago with Alzheimer's disease and now all those troubles with his care came to my mind.

I drove almost 200 kilometres to her and got her to the doctor's. My mother said that she could not remember things. I had recognised she did not know how to buy food or cook and she was not able to handle money. She was suspicious of neighbours ('stealing my newspaper', 'watching me going to the chemist's', 'stealing my roses from my back yard'). The doctor wrote a referral to the hospital for further investigation. We were told the waiting list for the hospital would be quite long.

I made a phone call to the social worker and asked if there was a day group for the people with such difficulties as my mother had. I was thinking that if she was in a day programme she would be able to live on her own for some months longer. I also asked if a home helper would visit her in the evening to help her with bathing, taking her medicine and going to bed.

The social worker was friendly but she explained that there were no day groups for older persons with dementia or other services like that in the village where my mother lived. The only place for getting help was an in-patient ward in the local health centre. However, she did not need hospital care and that would be the wrong place for her. Another possibility could be a group home run by a private organisation 30 kilometres away from my mother's home. However, there were no openings and a long waiting list. The only help the social worker could offer was visits of a home helper once a day and a warm meal on weekdays transported by a taxi driver. I felt desperate.

Summer 07 – Diagnosis
In July, after waiting for half a year, my mother saw the neurologist who told us the diagnosis: Alzheimer's disease. We were told that it could not be predicted how it would progress. She started the medication. I tried to see her as often as possible – almost every weekend. I noticed my mother did not remember to eat the meals and the taxi driver had no time to help her to eat. She was crying a lot and asked if I could live with her. But I have my family, two teenagers and a cat, who needed me as well; and I could not leave my job. I talked with my mother and we decided to put her on the waiting list for the group home.

December 07 – Non-institutional care
On Christmas morning my mother had a minor brain infarct (a stroke). Her walking and speaking were slightly damaged. But that was not the worst thing. The hospital was full of patients, and my mother's bed was

often in the day room or in a corridor. After a couple of weeks in hospital she, in a way, had lost her mind: she did not know who she was, or where she lived and she was very anxious about that. Anyway, she was sent home.

By Easter I was exhausted. I called the social worker who was the head of the older people's care services, the district nurse, the doctor, even the local politicians, and I tried to explain to them that my mother was not able to live alone. I asked why the municipal administration does not take responsibility for old, helpless people who have worked for tens of years and paid taxes believing they will get help when they need it. I was told that a person's own home is the best place for an old person – that is the strategy of the Ministry of Social and Health Care, too. I realised there were only two options: in-patient care in the hospital, which was not a realistic choice in this case, or staying at home with care that was not enough in her situation.

After all, she had a care package that consisted of meals-on-wheels, visits for medication twice a day and the alarm system that would give a signal if she pressed an alarm button or if she went out the front door. Now she was imprisoned in her own home. The care package was a combination of both municipal and private help. There were four people visiting her including a 'watch person' in case of emergencies. They changed according to the working timetable and shifts and stayed from one minute (the taxi-driver bringing the meal) to 30 minutes (if the home helper assisted her in taking a shower and going to bed).

One day a neighbour called me: 'Your mother is standing by the window and crying: Who has stolen my home? Where has my home gone?' A week ago she was standing on the balcony shouting for help as she did not know how to enter the room even though the door was open. A day after that, the children of the next door neighbour found her standing on the street wearing a bathrobe – she had gone out to find her lost home. So the alarm system did not work perfectly and she never learned how to press the alarm button . . .

August 08 – Institutional care
Finally, after waiting a year, my mother got a place in a group home run by a private organisation. She felt secure there and was doing better in many ways. However, one thing was not good in the group home, namely, there was a lack of staff. I found out that people living there had to stay inside every day. Outdoor recreation was totally dependent on the goodwill of visitors. In addition, due to lack of staff, all residents had to go to bed very early, at 19.00 hours, before the night nurse started her shift. If my mother said she did not want to go to bed so early the nurse

gave her a sleeping pill. I understood that happened because there was only one practical nurse taking care of 20 old people. She simply could not manage her work alone. So when visiting there I tried also to help other old people in whatever ways I could: I read them newspapers aloud, I talked with them, I helped them to have a glass of water, and so on.

In November I got a phone call from the social worker: my mother was going to be placed in another institution. The local authority had made a contract with a new service supplier. I had no choice but to complain about the decision. I was shocked. My mother had just learned to know her own room and her own bed, she had a friend from childhood with whom she shared the room. And now that the process was starting again, I guessed that it would be much more difficult for my mother than it was some months ago in the first group home.

Commentary 1

AIRA VANHALA

The Finnish welfare system

This case needs to be understood in the context of the history and current state of the welfare system in Finland. Social welfare services and benefits in Finland are based on the Nordic welfare state model with the ideal of universal services, based on principles of equality and justice. The public sector (the national state and the local authority) is responsible for providing and organising welfare services to meet the needs of citizens. The system is financed by local tax revenues paid by both individuals and local enterprises. Good levels of welfare services have enhanced the opportunities for women to enter into the labour market and the proportion of working women is traditionally high.

The Finnish welfare model was developed after the Second World War, during the period of reconstruction. Now, at the beginning of the twenty-first century, the situation in society is crucially different. The welfare state is facing severe problems because of the ageing population, increasing needs for welfare services, the decreasing rate of employment and tax revenues and global financial problems. With a neo-liberal ideology in the ascendant, the 'new public management' was introduced into the public sector to solve the financial problems. This is characterised by outsourcing of services, competition, a supply–demand model, cost effectiveness, a concern for productivity and an increasing transfer of responsibility for care to service users and their families.

The case in context

This case highlights the consequences of the new way of allocating resources for an individual service user and her carer in rural Finland. Here distances are large and in remote parts of the country the density of population is very low, 17.4 inhabitants per square kilometre on average. On the other hand, 1.5 million out of a total population of 5.3 million live in the capital region. There have been big changes in the country after the Second World War. The sense of community is far from what it used to be. Families have only one or two children, who tend to move to big cities for work. So it is challenging for people to have to turn to voluntary work or entrepreneurship or care given by the family, which are seen as new ways to organise welfare services.

In September 2009 reports about the situation relating to care for older people were given by provincial governments in Finland to the Parliamentary Ombudsman. According to these reports, there were lots of problems in municipalities. So the case of Maria presented here is not at all an exceptional one. The problems have been discussed for years in the media and amongst the politicians before the elections. All the same, almost nothing has been done to make things better.

We should not point the finger only at the attitudes of the staff in the institutions. The crucial factor is the decision-making about resources. And there are always values behind those decisions. Finland has proceeded strongly towards a meritocracy during the last decade. It indicates that the state's responsibility for the comprehensive welfare of citizens has disappeared. There is no 'social policy' in the sense in which the concept was used during the 1970s and 1980s. Instead, the strategy is nowadays based on the profitable functions of different levels of organisations. Comprehensive care of the elderly has been split into various types of services and each of them has its price. The local authority makes a contract with a service supplier for a certain period, for example, for two years. Now that this new model has been implemented in Finland for some years, it can be seen that it does not always direct the decision-making towards the quality of service or the needs of a service user, but towards the price.

Ethical issues and dilemmas

This case highlights sharply a range of policy-related questions about whose responsibility it is to provide care for older people (the state, family, or both); what should be the standards of care for older people in terms of preserving and respecting their dignity and quality of life; what are the rights of older people and families to state-provided care; and how can the increasing burden of caring for older people be distributed fairly between generations, families and taxpayers in the light of other priorities (such as child care, education, leisure provision).

In this case, the daughter clearly believed that her mother had a right to high quality state-provided care, having paid her taxes over many years in the expectation of receiving services in old age. Although at one point Maria asks her daughter if she can come and live with her, the daughter felt this was impossible because she could not leave her own family, job and other commitments. This was not really considered as a serious option, and certainly not as a duty or a necessity. The possibility of Maria living with her daughter and family was not mentioned. This case is clearly located in a paradigm that regards the care of the elderly as a state responsibility and places a high value on the independence of daughters and sons to pursue a career and live in independent family homes.

The case of Maria highlights clearly the difficulties for service users and carers in participating in their own care plans. Although the daughter was thought to participate in her mother's care, neither she nor Maria herself seems to have played any role in planning and implementing Maria's care. They were not heard in setting the aims, choosing the means of support or following the implementation of services.

It has been said that 'the structure gives results'. The prevailing strategy in Finland emphasises economic values and has brought changes in the structure of the professional staff. In Maria's case there were no social care workers or social pedagogues working in older people's care. The only professional representing social expertise was the manager of the care of the elderly in the local authority. She was not working closely with service users and so would not have had a great impact on the everyday practice in care units.

We know that the most costly part of older people's care is the staff. So organisations tend to save costs by employing as few workers as possible. Practical nurses, who comprise the majority of the staff, have to manage in under-resourced units day after day. There may be only one worker on the night shift and 20–30 more or less restless older people. This means that they cannot work in the way they know would be right and ethical. They have time to change incontinence pads only twice a day; they have to tie some of the most restless people to the bed in order to prevent them from hurting others or themselves; they have to give sleeping pills, and so on.

Now we come to the important question: What are the basic needs of a person, even though he or she is old, and even if he or she cannot express his or her wishes? Is outdoor recreation a basic need? What about social interaction and communication with other people? In everyday practice in older people's care it seems that human dignity consists of eating, sleeping and hygiene. Is that the picture of a good life? Would you like to have that kind of life when old?

The manager of elderly care was a professional social worker. However, she did not have much to offer when the daughter asked for help for her mother. She opted out of responsibility, pleading local and governmental strategies relating to older people's care. We can ask if the social worker could and should highlight the needs of older people more strongly to the stakeholders. Armed with that information the stakeholders could consider other options, not only that of a simple choice between either staying at home or staying at an in-patient ward in the health centre.

Lack of resources and the strict policy based on the idea of living at home are not a good combination in this case, or in many other similar cases. This case raises a number of issues and questions, including:

* How to solve the dilemma between the quality of services and the demand for cost-effectiveness and productivity.
* What is the ethical responsibility of the organisation for all members of the community? How do you balance resource allocation between all service users with declining resources?
* How to sustain the stakeholders' interest in ethical questions, and how to keep up the conversation on ethical values in organisations.

Aira Vanhala, M.Sc., is Senior Lecturer at Oulu University of Applied Sciences, Finland. Her special areas of interest are social work methodology and social policy.

Commentary 2

HIROSHI KOSAKA

In this case, the structural cause of the problem about the provision of care is the gap between the wishes of the carer (the daughter), who is acting as the voice of the service user (the mother), and the services arranged. However, there are many other factors involved in this case. In the following commentary, I will summarise the situation and indicate some key features of the case. Then I will reorder these points and consider the common ethical issues.

At the beginning, the daughter hoped that it would be possible for her mother to attend a day group, and for home helpers to visit her in her home. However, this was not possible, and her mother's condition deteriorated more and more. The daughter did not know what to do in this situation. In the region where her mother lived there were no day groups. As a structural feature of the welfare system, this can be characterised as *the problem of regional gaps in services.*

Although the daughter described the social worker with whom she spoke as friendly, the social worker proposed that her mother should just receive a visit from a home helper once a day and a warm meal once on weekdays. Whatever the social worker may have felt about this offer of services, in these circumstances it seems that she (or he) could only play *the role of 'gatekeeper'* in this system.

In July, the progress of the mother's Alzheimer's disease was reported to be unpredictable by the doctor. The daughter was not able to come and live with her mother. She decided to put her mother's name on the waiting list for a place in a group home. Nevertheless, we could probably regard this as a decision made reluctantly by the daughter. We can deduce that the level of nursing care provided in the hospital (experienced when her mother had a cerebral infarction in December) was not adequate due to the large number of patients. The exhausted daughter called the social worker, the district nurse, the doctor and the local politicians and appealed for their help in the current situation. This *insistence on citizenship* was perfectly justified. However, she was made to recognise that she had no alternative but to choose between the two options for her mother (going to hospital or staying in her own home), because the authorities pushed the responsibility back onto her as the daughter *by using government policy as a shield.*

After all, her mother had got a care package, including an alarm system. The purpose of an alarm system is to secure the safety of service users. However, only if we look at the situation from the viewpoint of the service user can we judge whether or not this service is really adequate or useful. Such a service can be *interpreted as better or worse depending on the service user's particular circumstances and by taking the service user's perspective.* Even from the perspective of a layperson, this care package is *obviously an insufficient service* for a progressively deteriorating Alzheimer's disease patient. As a result, the alarm system was not only insufficient but also *might risk causing an accident.*

Her mother was finally able to enter the group home after a year. Her living conditions became better. However, because of staff shortages the people living there could not go outdoors. The situation in the group home was such that the daughter found herself also looking after other elderly people. Then, just when her mother was becoming familiar with the home and her condition began to show signs of improvement, she was transferred to another facility. The comments made by the daughter at the end of this case suggest fears of her mother's *deterioration caused by the so-called 'relocation effect'*.

I would now like to draw attention to several important points about this case:

1   The overall levels of provision available in the welfare system and regional gaps in services.
2   A social worker acting as a 'gatekeeper'.
3   A difficult decision urged on a service user and her carer.
4   A situation in which the citizenship of a service user is not respected.
5   A level of service that leads to a worsening of the condition of the service user.

Three ethical considerations emerge from these points. To begin with, there is *the issue of the system*. A welfare system is not adequate if it does not place the needs of service users at its centre. The defining feature of welfare policy is the satisfaction of individuals' needs for welfare. In this sense, it is different from other policy areas, such as economic policy. Therefore, it is important that any welfare system provides a variety of services so that it can respond to different needs. However, there are financial limits to the levels of services that can be provided. On the one hand, it is difficult to implement welfare as a practical economic policy (which also links with the issue of variations in the regional distribution of services as noted in point 1 above). On the other hand, in spite of economic considerations, it is important that there should be fairness in the distribution of services in the welfare system. The achievement of social justice is important for the welfare of society. We should be able to say that we will construct the welfare system for that purpose. At the very least, it is important to enhance the welfare system on the basis of promoting social justice.

Secondly, there is *the issue of the role of the social work practitioner*. One of the important functions required of a social worker is not to take on a 'gatekeeper' role, but rather to act as an advocate on behalf of the service user (see point 2). For this reason, the social worker occasionally engages in social action. Indeed, the social worker's supportive response can be grounded in an inner human impulse when confronted with other people who are vulnerable. However, the social worker is also located as a bureaucrat within an organisation and offers social support to vulnerable people as part of her or his professional work. These are two equally important dimensions of the practice of the social worker, and it is not desirable for either of them to become dominant at the expense of the other.

Thirdly, there is the question of *the relationship between the welfare system and practice*. It is true that the welfare system provides the support given by the social worker. However, if the management of the system proceeds too much in the direction of managerialism, the social worker will become a 'gatekeeper' – because an excessive strengthening of operational management is connected directly with the worker's functional management. As a result, a situation arises where the service required by the service user does not exist; instead the service user is expected to fit into the available services (see point 3). This is a case of misplaced priorities, based on a misunderstanding of the purpose of the welfare system. The system seems to exist for its own sake, and neither the service user nor the social worker feature on the horizon (see point 4).

The policy maker should consider this situation. As the social worker is in the frontline, s/he is likely to be able to understand a lot about what happens in practice. It should be recognised that if the service fails to meet the wishes and needs of the service user, then it is to be expected that the condition of the service user will deteriorate (see point 5). On this basis, it is important that social workers and other professionals propose changes to the national and local government policies and practices and also help stimulate and support citizens' movements campaigning for social change.

Finally, according to the philosopher Emmanuel Levinas (1989), at the heart of ethics is a meeting place where one person encounters the face of the other, who makes a call or a summons. In this case, we (the readers) encounter the 'face' of the carer who was misled by the system. But the professionals in this case did not seem to respond to the faces of the service user and the carer, whose particular features, emotions and desires were excluded. This encapsulates the deep ethical problem that lies at the core of this case: the inability of professionals genuinely to meet the mother and daughter face to face and respond to their actual demands.

Reference

Levinas, E. (1989) 'Ethics as first philosophy', translated by Seán Hand, in S. Hand (ed.) *The Levinas Reader*, Oxford: Blackwell.

Hiroshi Kosaka is Associate Professor in Welfare Sociology in the Faculty of Community Policy at Aichi Gakusen University, Japan.

Questions for discussion about Case 6.3

1 What do you think should be the role of the state in the provision of care for older people? What is the policy and practice in your own area/country?
2 One of the key ethical principles of the health and social care professions is to respect and promote the dignity of service users. What do you think would count as 'dignity' for Maria and her daughter in this case?
3 The social professions frequently operate in situations of resource constraints and inadequate services. What can they do to publicise and challenge the reasons for these situations?

Case study 6.4

Case 6.4 Maintaining professional integrity in an area of conflict: working with a sexually abused girl in the Occupied Palestinian Territories

Introduction

This case is situated in East Jerusalem in an area which has been occupied by Israel since 1967 and is under Israeli law. There have been two major uprisings (Intifada) against the occupation by the indigenous Palestinian Arab population. The conflict is enduring with no real prospects of a durable peace settlement. The occupation has been characterised by a major growth in Israeli settlements in the Occupied Palestinian Territories (OPT), home demolitions, land confiscation and the construction of a separation wall around Palestinian communities. The movement of Palestinians within the Occupied Territories is also severely restricted and there are high levels of poverty and unemployment. Within the Palestinian community, cooperation with the Israeli occupying power can be seen as collaboration with the enemy and those suspected of this may be subject to community punishment. Palestinian social workers have to be very careful not to be seen to cooperate with the Israelis against their own traditions and culture.

The legal jurisdiction is complex. Some areas, such as East Jerusalem, are fully under occupation and Israeli jurisdiction. Israel has a well-developed child protection system. Under the Penal Law, 1977 (chapter 10, section 5(1)) every individual is under obligation to report to the authorities a suspicion that a child is suffering from neglect, abandonment, assault or physical, mental or sexual abuse by a parent or guardian. Failure to report constitutes a criminal offence, with more severe maximum penalties imposed for breach of this obligation on professionals such as doctors, nurses, people who work in the education system, social workers and psychologists.

In other areas, namely the West Bank and Gaza, the Palestinian Authority has limited self-determination and legislative authority. Within these areas a child protection system is being developed and the Palestinian Law No. (7) of 2004, *Concerning the Children*, which covers child protection and abuse, is yet to be fully implemented. Social services, the police and the judiciary are currently developing procedures and processes. The system is still in its infancy and it will take time for this to be fully accepted. In developing this system consultation meetings were held with stakeholders in local communities. Though the new child protection system allows for children to be removed from the family home, there is a strong emphasis on seeking support for the young person from other members of the family and local community. Only when this fails will the option of removing a child from the home be considered. However, at present, any removal of a female child is likely to have a negative impact on the child herself in her community of origin.

Social workers have to be very careful if and when they have to move a child and they need to do this with the support of the extended family/community as far as possible otherwise they as social workers would not be able to function in the society as they would lose community consent to their role. They do not yet have the support of the community in these matters. Palestinian communities are close knit and are characterised by large extended families and collective solidarity. Within segments of the community, behaviour which is seen to bring 'dishonour' to the family can be severely sanctioned and so called 'honour' killings are not unknown.

School-based social workers/counsellors are the largest group of psycho-social workers working with children in the OPT. They are employed by the Palestinian Authority and by the United Nations Relief and Works Agency (UNRWA) who have provided services to Palestinian refugees and their families since 1948 from the area which is now the State of Israel and who have no direct relationship with the Israeli authorities.

The case

Rana, a Palestinian girl aged 14 from East Jerusalem, told her school social worker that her father was sexually abusing her. The social worker obtained Rana's permission to inform the head teacher of the school and Rana's mother. Together they decided how to talk to Rana's father and put in place a child protection plan. The mother confronted her husband. He did not deny that he had abused his daughter. The family had a room which was separate from their main house. The father agreed to stay in this room. He was not to enter the family home unless his wife was present and he gave up his keys to the house. Rana was given a key to her room so she could lock herself in. She was also given counselling and assertiveness training. The cooperation between the mother, the head teacher, school social worker and Rana was successful. Rana's academic performance, self-esteem and confidence improved. Her father kept to his promise. Knowledge of what happened was kept within the small circle of the professionals, the girl and her mother and father.

This case should been reported to the Israeli authorities as she was a resident of East Jerusalem. There is generally a strong reluctance to report issues to the Israeli authorities and in this case the social worker and head teacher's position was to avoid such reporting if at all possible. Given that such reporting is mandatory and non-reporting is a criminal offence, any decision which goes against the legal requirement carries a degree of risk for all involved. In this case, this was weighed against the possible outcomes of making such a report. Had it been reported, the girl might have been removed from her family and placed in a children's home under Israeli supervision while the situation was being investigated. There is community suspicion of these institutions and it is rumoured that girls who are placed in such institutions get involved in drugs, prostitution or are even induced to inform on their communities. In Palestinian communities people know each other's business and rumours become facts. No one checks to find out if there is truth in these rumours or not. People just repeat them. Had Rana been removed she might never have been able to return to 'normal' community life. The case would have become community knowledge. This could have meant that Rana might also have been at risk of being killed (as she was living in a so-called 'honour' community). She would not have been able to complete her schooling, work or even marry. Furthermore, her father would have been arrested and imprisoned. As the main wage earner for a large family, the family would have been ruined socially and economically, the former being more important culturally. The community would know the reason for the arrest. Not only would Rana have been affected, but also her sisters' and brothers' life chances would have been impacted negatively. In this case, the outcome was positive. In a situation where the father had denied the allegation and refused to cooperate, the situation would have become more complex and the social worker, head teacher and mother would have had to consider alternative courses of action. It is currently likely that this would not have involved informing the Israeli authorities, but other informal means to protect Rana without disclosing the situation to others would have been sought. In the view of the professionals involved it was felt that it will take a long time for Palestinian children to be seen only as victims of abuse and to be able to recover positively within their community of origin.

Commentary 1

MAHMOUD BAIDOUN AND JANE LINDSAY

The main ethical problems in this case stem from the question of whether or not to obey the law, which requires the school social worker to report the alleged abuse. This case is complicated in that the law in question is one imposed by an occupying power (Israel), whose remit is not accepted, but is enforced, in the area in which Rana lives, the disputed territory of East Jerusalem. This is further compounded by the fact that Rana's community and school align themselves with the Occupied Palestinian Territories whose relevant legal provisions (the Palestinian Law No. (7) of 2004, *Concerning the Children*) are only in the process of being introduced. If the school social worker was to adhere to Palestinian Law, she would be required to report Rana's case to the child protection social worker in the region, conduct an initial interview with the child in the school to listen to her story, and assess whether Rana was in danger or potential danger. A Palestinian child protection social worker has the legal right to decide to take the child away from his/her family within 48 hours if the social worker believes that there is a threat to the young person's life. There are considerable similarities in both Israeli and Palestinian child protection legislation, both of which are concerned to protect the child and deal with the perpetrator of abuse in a way that safeguards not only the child concerned but also other children within the family network. Both have mandatory requirements to report abuse.

Professional social workers should normally work within the law. The issue is what is the ethical justification for this social worker choosing not to report the case to the relevant authorities? It would seem probable that the legitimacy of the Israeli legal authority is questioned by the actors in this case. However, the decision-making outlined above does not merely seem to be located within the framework of civil disobedience in times of war. Having decided not to report to the Israeli authorities, should the social worker not then have reported to the Palestinian Authority? The social worker and the family and school might have accepted the legitimacy of the Palestinian Authority, but it appears that the remit of the Authority in the geographical location is very limited, or perhaps non-existent. Further, given that the legal frameworks for child protection are at an early stage of development, it is possible that there may have been a lack of confidence in these systems – another legitimacy gap. It would appear from the description that the school social worker took the view in this instance that it was morally permissible not to obey the law because of the weight of the consequences that might occur as a result of taking such an action within the cultural context. Her actions were essentially contextually located and pragmatic.

In Palestine, for cases like Rana's, an exception is sometimes applied to legislative frameworks to help save the girl from a fate worse than death. Although school counsellors and social workers are trained to deal with such cases in accordance with the child law and child protection system, nevertheless, sexual abuse has to be assessed and dealt with in accordance with the victim's circumstances and wishes, as Rana's case clearly demonstrates. The protection process is very sensitive in the Palestinian context, and depends on a Code of Ethics and Practice to ensure different principles such as confidentiality, victim safety, respect and acceptance, and the right to get access to the services for rehabilitation.

Decision-making that involves not working within the law in such cases carries clear risks, and raises the question of whether it is dangerous to depart from the law. Setting aside the legal penalties school social workers may face in both jurisdictions for failing to report, this social school worker appears to have taken action to spread, and possibly to reduce, the risk by involving others (the head teacher and Rana's mother) and developing a 'community of care'. Taking these factors into account, the actions of the school social worker and her colleagues could be argued to be morally defensible (although the question remains about whether the father was justly treated within these arrangements). The school social worker appears to have been motivated by care for the young person. She was working, possibly instinctively, from a virtue ethics perspective, balancing rules and consequences and employing an understanding of what Rana needed to protect her immediately and to enable her to function well in her community and society in future.

However, we might judge that the father's behaviour is highly likely to be compulsive and he may have no control over his conduct. This means that the solution of keeping the father in a separate room as mentioned in the case study would not be realistic at all, as he might try to sexually abuse Rana again, or her sisters, if she has any. Furthermore, without individual intervention, Rana may well continue to suffer from flashbacks of the critical events and therefore may never get her life back again. Sexual abuse is a complex matter and needs joint efforts from a specialist professional team. If this case had been dealt with through a child protection referral system and had been taken through the recognised stages, then it is highly likely that a decision would have been made to remove the source of danger, the father, from the home. The *fadiha* (social scandal) issue should be considered, but not at the expense of the victim.

We need to strike a balance between protecting the child according to the referral system and treating each case as unique. This is the kind of debate we should have in order to really protect children in Palestine and that is exactly the goal of the new referral system that has been developed.

Mahmoud Baidoun Ph.D. Res. is Senior Trainer, Trauma Psychologist and Clinical Supervisor at the Mental Health Programme, Centre for Continuing Education, Birzeit University, Palestine. He has played a leading role in developing the new child protection referral system in Palestine.

Jane Lindsay is Deputy Head, School of Social Work, Kingston University/St George's, University of London. She is from Northern Ireland, and is a social worker and lecturer. From 1997 to 2009 she was the independent evaluator *pro bono* of schools counselling and professional supervision programmes offered by Birzeit University in the Occupied Palestinian Territories.

Commentary 2

DAVID N. JONES

This case highlights some of the core ethical tensions for social workers working in or with public (state managed) social welfare systems, especially the tension between individual, community and state interests. There are stark (and in global terms rare) issues of choice about cooperation with the civil authority during territorial occupation – but similar issues can arise in seemingly more stable situations.

Respect for law – the nature of civil authority

In this case there is a clear legal procedure requiring the reporting of suspected child abuse to civil authorities, namely Israeli social services. The rationale for mandatory reporting (implying breach of confidentiality) is that: there are reasonable grounds to suspect that a serious offence has been committed which must be investigated; the offence is likely to be repeated unless challenged (based on research evidence and experience); a vulnerable person (the child) will suffer lasting personal trauma unless the crime is stopped; and others may be at risk. Therefore proactive intervention is required to protect the child (and by implication other children) and provide therapeutic support. Public agencies in most situations also recognise that they face major public criticism if they ignore situations of risk which are later exposed (a defensive response).

This rationale is fatally undermined, in the view of the social workers in this case, because the civil authority is not respected or trusted to act in the best interests of the child, the family and the community, because it is seen as the agent of an occupying power. The consequences for the child of reporting are seen as worse than not reporting. There also appear to be alternative strategies which better serve the common good. The value placed on the individual welfare of the young person and the importance of 'community' thus outweigh the significance of legal duties. Such choices are not theoretical. Social workers (and others) in such situations face substantial personal risk, whatever choices they make, including risk of criminal prosecution and imprisonment.

In the United Kingdom context, social workers in Northern Ireland during 'The Troubles' (a period of violent conflict at its most intense between 1968–1998) often had to negotiate 'permission' from Republicans to enter certain areas to enforce child protection procedures. They would sometimes be accompanied by paramilitaries. They also knew that, after they departed, there was often a risk that the paramilitaries would undertake their own justice against alleged abusers, such as 'kneecapping' (shooting in the knee) and severe beatings of members. The decision to investigate, therefore, carried unpredictable consequences. Social workers managed to retain the confidence of all the main political groups during this period, reflecting their skill in avoiding becoming identified with one side or the other, in contrast to the police. In the case of Northern Ireland, social workers also adapted allegiance to civil authority to local political realities.

In practice this dilemma is frequently present for social workers in a range of less conflictual situations. First nation and indigenous communities have experienced decades of intervention, removing children into state sponsored alternative care leaving them alienated from families, communities and heritage, sometimes emotionally damaged and in many cases seriously abused. Many social workers are also concerned at the failure of public care systems to provide good enough care, leaving the unanswered question, 'Will the child do better in care?'

Rights of the child

All actors in this situation recognise the need to respect the rights of a young person to be free of abuse. In this case, the social worker sought the girl's permission to inform others. In some countries, the evidence of a crime and the need for protection overrides the young person's right to confidentiality and to have a say in what happens. Yet many young people say they do not want intervention and family break-up; they 'just want the abuse to stop'. In this case, the young person is given considerable 'rights' within the home (such as the right to lock her bedroom door), which is unusual. It is arguable that the right of a young person to family life and to the opportunity of a 'normal' upbringing is given significant respect in this case, but only at the risk of undermining another right – to be free from further abuse – which could be forfeited in the short term. Social work frequently involves a balance of rights.

Rights of the parents

The parents have rights to due process and family life, unless this is overridden by crime or other major factors. In this case, the mother is given additional authority within the household, although with no real power to enforce this if the father breaks the agreement. The father agrees to live in a separated room and not to enter the house. This solution allows the parents to continue to care for their daughter despite the abuse. In all child-abuse situations, social workers are seeking to mediate often conflicting rights and principles, usually aiming to favour the individual rights of the child. In more communitarian environments, the individual rights of the child may be seen as subservient to the greater good of the community.

Use of research – risk from perpetrators

This case example poses an ethical question about the use of research to inform practice. There is substantial evidence that male perpetrators in Western cultures are more likely to continue abusing than to stop when challenged, even where there is a formal agreement about such things as not being in the same room as the victim. In this case, the professional's choice to leave the young person at home with the father living in the same environment, albeit in an outside room, involves some risk for her. However, the case suggests that handling the problem went well and there was no further abuse and the young person gained in self respect. This points to the complex ethical issues concerning the use of research in social work practice. Research generally tends to point to possibilities (or even probabilities) but not certainties. In practice, a judgement has to be made about the differing level of risk in every case. It seems probable that explicit reference to findings from research will increasingly be found in case recordings and also in case studies like this.

Role-perspective of workers

The social workers have an ethical choice to make in situations of occupation or civil conflict – a choice which confronts all social workers involved in public systems, namely whether to obey laws and employer instructions about dealing with people or whether to put the perceived interests and rights of the individual before all else. In this case, social workers and teachers took significant personal risks to respect the rights of the young person and the family to family life.

David N. Jones is a registered social worker with 35 years' experience in child protection work and national policy roles in the UK. As President of the International Federation of Social Workers (2006–2010) he witnessed social work practice in many countries. His doctoral thesis was on the evaluation and inspection of social work. He has published, and lectures, on social work practice and management.

Questions for discussion about Case 6.4

1 What issues does this case raise about the role of social workers in areas of conflict, especially territories that are under occupation?
2 Do you think the social worker and teacher in this case were right to deal with it themselves by working with the family, without going through the official channels? Is there a difference

between judging a decision or action to be legally right and judging it to be ethically right?

3   The outcomes for the young woman are reported to have been good in this case. If the outcomes had been bad (if the abuse had continued or she had become pregnant) would this influence your view about whether the decisions and actions of the social worker and teacher were ethically right?

Working with cases and commentaries

Sarah Banks and Kirsten Nøhr

Introduction

The aim of this chapter is to provide materials for students, practitioners and teachers to use in undertaking further study on ethical issues and dilemmas in social work. In the previous chapters of the book cases are grouped together under themes, and each case is accompanied by two commentaries and a set of questions for discussion. The first part of this chapter comprises six cases from different parts of the world, without commentaries, that are not grouped or interpreted in any way. These can then be used as a focus for discussion and interpretation by the readers themselves and as a basis for readers to write their own commentaries. In the second part of the chapter we offer some exercises based around using cases and commentaries in learning and teaching.

Ethical difficulties occur in practice when social workers are working with individuals or groups in institutional or more 'private' settings. There is usually a necessity to act – in the immediacy of the situation and over the course of time. This involves what Schön (1991) calls 'reflection-in-action' – making assessments and evaluations in the course of doing the work about what is going on and what to do next.

A different kind of reflection comes afterwards: 'reflection-on-action'. As can be seen in many of the cases presented in this book, the memory of what happened, and the question of whether the actions taken and outcomes achieved were right or wrong, good or bad, can stay in the minds of social workers for many years. The process of reflecting on a case, past event or situation and carrying its features in our memories is an important source of learning for social workers and other professionals. Reflection, reflexivity and dialogue are key concepts in the context of difficult ethical situations and decisions. Social workers' choices and actions are always embedded in particular political, cultural and social contexts. Being aware of one's own background, identity, position and power (for example, gender, ethnicity, job status) is part of what is meant by reflexivity and is a crucial element in any ethical evaluation or action (Fook and Askeland 2006; Taylor 2006).

After an event or decision we frequently ask ourselves questions like: 'What actually happened?', 'Why did it happen?', 'Why were certain decisions made?', 'Who was responsible?', 'What was my role?', 'What power did I have?' and 'How could I have acted differently?' These questions are open to interpretation. Interpretations can be made on the basis of ethical theories, but the social and cultural background and personal experience of the interpreter also play a crucial role, as we can see from the different commentaries in the previous chapters.

The cases in this book are stories told about actions that happened in real life. But when 'reality' is told or written down, it is always seen through the eyes of the storyteller, and only a selection of details is included. There will always be more behind the words. We might say that a qualified reflection has to take place in the space between the words and the action. In the cases that follow we invite readers to interrogate critically the assemblage of 'facts', ideas, thoughts, judgements and feelings included in each case and to examine the way the narrator tells the story – with a view to offering their own analysis and interpretations, and perhaps even writing commentaries themselves.

Cases without commentaries

The cases that follow are all about real situations, some written from personal experience, others based on accounts given by social workers or abstracted from the professional casework of an association.

Taking money from a dubious source: a dilemma for a social worker in China

Introduction

This case is about a dilemma faced by a social worker in China. China is an extremely complex country. On the one hand, China's traditional political system, social structure, customs and culture have been radically changed in recent years (since 1949 when the Communist system was established); on the other hand, a new system of social rules in China has not been completely established. In these circumstances, China's social work has many different characteristics when compared with the work in other countries. Firstly, this field is mainly controlled by the government, thus almost all of the current social workers and service providers have governmental backgrounds. Secondly, social workers and related institutions do not have sufficient finance and decision-making power to assist service users. Thirdly, many social workers and officers working in public welfare institutions have not been professionally trained, and simply conduct the work based on their own judgement and experiences.

The case

Due to limited finances and decision-making power, China's social workers and related welfare officers sometimes need to seek assistance from government departments and businesses. During their careers, social workers and welfare officers may face certain kinds of ethical dilemmas, of which this case is one example.

Several years ago, Mr Chen, a social worker, was in charge of seeking financial support for children in low-income families. He worked in a large city for a non-governmental organisation (NGO) that provided support to children who were homeless and from low-income families. Through a government officer's introduction, Mr Chen met an entrepreneur, Mr Li, who owned a large business with a high reputation in the city. Mr Li expressed the following sentiments: 'I also experienced a period of poor life. I know how those poor children are feeling, so I will help them.' After a short conversation with Mr Chen, Mr Li promised to provide sufficient finance for 10 children, covering their school tuition fees, general living expenditure, and so on. In fact, Mr Li ended up supporting at least 30 children. Besides this, Mr Li always assisted Mr Chen in working with those children. He was involved in the process of teaching them how to be responsible people in society, encouraging them to be stronger, and providing some simple emotional therapies, and so on. With Mr Li's support, the conditions of many children were obviously improved and their prospects became more optimistic than before. Mr Chen and his colleagues all considered that Mr Li was a responsible and respectful man.

Unfortunately, as time went by, Mr Chen gradually found out that Mr Li's business was in severe violation of the country's laws. What was worse, Mr Li was suspected of being involved in illegally regulating the market. Although these behaviours may not appear to hurt anybody directly, obviously they can cause negative influences in society. According to China's law, Mr Chen has an obligation to report these criminal issues to the relevant government departments. However, if he did this, those children might lose their schooling, comfortable accommodation, and, above all, a real hero in their hearts. Mr Chen felt confused about what he should do.

As William Shakespeare (the English dramatist and poet) said, a person may act in many different roles in society. Mr Li was playing a role as a generous and caring benefactor, whilst at the same time he was engaging in illegal business practices. This case is not a rare phenomenon in China. Because of the high levels of competition and the special situation in China, it is not easy to judge when a person or action is right or wrong.

Case 7.2

Maintaining professional secrecy: a French ethical situation

Introduction

The professional association for social workers in France (Association Nationale des Assistantes de Service Social, ANAS) represents the profession and promotes social work values at all levels. One of the aims of the association is to clarify the values that underlie the interventions of social workers, in particular to assure service users the guarantee of common values of all social work professionals. ANAS supports all professionals who might have problems with their institution or with police services which are contrary to the professional ethical code. This case is an example of support given to a professional who was confronted with difficulties with a police service.

The case[1]

On 17th July 2007, a social worker, who was a member of the ANAS in Belfort (a town close to the Swiss and the German borders), was interrogated by the border police and put in custody. The social worker was based at a refuge for women who have been victims of violence (centre d'hébergement et de réinsertion pour les femmes battues). The social worker was reproached by the police for not having given the address of a particular woman who no longer had a valid residence permit allowing her to stay in France. This woman had stayed in the Centre where the professional was working. The woman had been beaten by her male companion and was put in a safe place by the social welfare organisation that employed the social worker. The social worker specified that she could not give the woman's address because she (the social worker) was subject to the rules of professional secrecy. In France, professional social workers are subject to a law that requires them not to reveal personal information about their clients. In responding to the request from the police officers, she would have committed an offence.

However, according to the police, this professional was also at risk of being sued for 'aiding illegal residency'. This regulation stipulates that a person who helps someone without official papers (an illegal resident) is committing an offence (a penal infringement).

However, in the view of ANAS, this situation was an infringement of human rights, as stipulated in international, regional, European and national conventions. Social workers have a function to help people, including adults and minors, French and foreigners, with or without papers. When they protect a beaten woman, or allow a pregnant woman to access care, or support a family that needs food, they are not assisting illegal residency, but rather supporting people's rights for a decent life.

ANAS gave its total support to this social worker. Indeed, social workers are required to maintain professional secrecy legally and professionally (as outlined in article L 411 of the Social Action and Families Code and article 226-13 of the Penal Code). If they have to answer to police inquiries they also have to keep silent about the private

1 This case was the subject of a presentation at a meeting organised at the DGAS (General Direction of Social Action) on 9th July 2009.

facts they get to know about within the framework of their profession. There is only a duty to speak if the person in question is in danger (article 226-14 of the Penal Code), which was obviously not the case in this situation. In addition, it is worth remembering that illegal residency is not one of the exemptions to professional secrecy contained in article 226-14 of the Penal Code.

ANAS supported this social worker, and the outcome was that the Prosecutor of the Belfort Republic did not pursue the case further.

Case 7.3

Institutional pressures and social work ethics: a case from Jamaica

Introduction

The Government of Jamaica has sought to honour its obligations as a signatory to the United Nations Convention on the Rights of the Child by enacting The Child Care and Protection Act[2] which introduces mandatory reporting of known or suspected cases of child abuse or neglect. The government did not simply pass this legislation, which prescribes relatively severe penalties for non-compliance, it also initiated the reform of the child protection system, established the Office of the Children's Registry to which reports of abuse should be made, and created the position of Children's Advocate. This is a type of ombudsperson who has a status equivalent to that of a High Court judge with powers to investigate any matter related to the welfare of children, especially those in the care of the state or receiving services from a public agency such as a school. Additionally the Jamaican Ministry of Education has revised its Education Regulations, to prohibit the use of corporal punishment in schools.

These measures have helped to increase the attention paid to the rights and treatment of children in Jamaica, both on the part of members of the public sector and the wider community. However, their consistent and successful implementation is undermined by a strong 'anti-informer' culture, where popular sentiment does not support individuals making reports about wrongdoing (whistle blowing), especially in situations where

2 Government of Jamaica (2004) The Child Care and Protection Act, available from www.cda.gov.jm/child_care_protection_act.php

the 'informer' (whistle blower) could suffer serious negative sanctions (including harm to one's career prospects, or even death in some cases). In addition, neither the new nor restructured child welfare and child protection agencies have been given adequate resources to carry out their work. Finally, while the legislation imposes penalties on civilians and members of designated professions such as teaching and social work, social work in Jamaica is not a protected profession, so there is no mechanism for dealing with cases of professional misconduct on the part of social workers.

The case[3]

Dr Glen Foster had successfully combined a career as a practitioner and social work educator for several years. He had pursued his social work training at university, both in Jamaica and in the United States. In both instances his courses had included content on social work ethics. Following graduation, the four years he spent in a Jamaican non-governmental community development agency inspired a passion for working with children as he encountered first-hand the abuse and deprivation that children living in the inner city experience. Returning to university overseas to do doctoral work, his dissertation on the impact of exposure to violence was the first of many studies he would produce over the next ten years. He also used the time abroad to take a number of short courses in therapeutic interventions with children who were victims of violence, and did an internship at a leading child welfare agency. When he returned home he easily got a job teaching in the social work programme at the university which was his alma mater and got involved in a church-sponsored project that provided services for vulnerable children referred by local schools and community organisations.

By the second year, Glen's colleagues began to have some concerns about the project, having heard that it sometimes bypassed the official child protection agencies. However, when they raised the issue with their colleague he argued that the official agencies took too long to respond to cases when they were reported. He added that in any event, having served on the committee to develop the procedures used by these very agencies, he made sure that project staff observed the relevant protocols.

The social work faculty members knew that heightened public awareness had given rise to many more cases of abuse coming to light. They

---

3 While this case is based on real events, certain aspects have been changed to protect the identity of the individuals and organisations that were actually involved.

realised that the graduate and undergraduate students who did their practicum with the project frequently worked many more hours than was required. They knew that despite Dr Foster's best efforts, the growing number of clients meant that he sometimes missed scheduled supervisory sessions with students. They were also unclear about the theoretical or empirical foundation of some of the treatment strategies used by Dr Foster and other members of the clinical team, although they wondered if this was due to their own lack of knowledge about the field. On the other hand, the project was one of the few settings in which students were able to receive the kind of exposure to a problem which was recognised nationally as being of critical importance. In fact it was a popular placement for students attracted by the nature of the work and Dr Foster's charismatic personality.

However, the Director of Field Education at the university became very concerned when she heard two graduate students in a seminar give a report on a case in which an eight-year-old child had been verbally and physically abused by a teacher. The students said that the only actions taken had been to arrange counselling for the child and a workshop on alternative methods of discipline for the teachers. In a meeting with the students following their seminar, the Director of Field Education enquired whether steps had also been taken to report the matter to the Children's Registry as was required by law. The students informed her that this action had not been taken and that Dr Foster had told them that this was not necessary because it was up to the school to make the necessary report. They admitted that they knew that in most cases no report was ever made, because the school authorities were reluctant to expose the school to the negative publicity that was often associated with matters of this nature. Despite this acknowledgement, and while expressing their own concerns about this and other aspects of their field experience, the students were clear that they were neither willing to make the reports themselves nor to participate in a meeting with their supervisor that the Field Education Director proposed.

Following the meeting, the Director contemplated her next steps. Previous efforts to deal with her colleague had not produced the desired change especially since involvement in the project was already earning kudos for him and, by association, for the university. The students' unwillingness to come forward meant that she would have little evidence to corroborate her own report; yet she kept thinking about the fact that the law mandated reporting on not just known but also suspected instances of impropriety. Was this such a case? What about the project's manager (who was not a trained social worker), or even the officials at the school the child attended? Did they have a greater responsibility to meet the requirements of the law? What about the implications for the credibility of the social work programme itself? Was it undermined by allowing this unsatisfactory state of affairs to continue?

Case 7.4

Between education and punishment: dilemmas for a Malaysian youth worker

Introduction

This case comes from a youth worker working for the Muslim Youth Movement of Malaysia (ABIM). ABIM is the leading Muslim youth organisation in Malaysia. In Malaysia there is a system of professional education and qualification for youth workers (organised by the government since 1997), but unfortunately it is not popular. ABIM is in the process of trying to develop training and qualifications and is playing a leading role in developing work with young people in Malaysia.

The case

Firdaus was a youth worker employed by ABIM in Malaysia. He developed an intervention initiative to solve disciplinary problems amongst students of a local secondary school who were regarded as 'hard core and problematic'. These students were young men who were aged 15–16 years old. The disciplinary problems consisted of truancy, fighting each other, smoking, gang-related violence and fighting with teachers. ABIM took responsibility to help the state government, especially the police, to reduce the incidence of crimes among the students. This was ABIM's first attempt to offer support to schools through the State Department of Education in solving disciplinary problems. ABIM staff had been involved in giving motivational talks to the students before, under the student development programme, but now they were extending their efforts to include intervention and eradication programmes.

Firdaus designed an intervention initiative which would involve bringing a cohort of these problematic students to what he and his colleagues described as 'hope city' (in fact a prison) for 'two days and one night'. They used the name 'hope city' to describe the prison, as they regarded it as probably the most efficacious tool for transforming the attitudes and behaviour of these students. At the beginning of the programme the terms 'hope city' and 'holiday' were intentionally used in discussing the trip with the students, as it was felt that if the students realised that they were to be taken to the prison, possibly they would not join the programme.

The main objective of this 'holiday' was to expose the students to the real and terrible life in prison, with the hope that through experiential learning this would help them to make transformational changes in their lives and encourage them to abstain from any acts that would eventually lead them to prison. The expectation was that the students would avoid committing further disciplinary problems and crimes in the school and start focusing on their studies. The reasoning behind this was that they would come to realise that if they continued with their ill-disciplined and criminal behaviour in the future, their next destination would definitely be prison.

Firdaus negotiated with the State Department of Education and got their agreement to bring a group of 39 problematic students to prison for the intervention initiative. ABIM managed to raise funds to bring all 39 students from the city where they were based, down to the south of Peninsular Malaysia – a journey of 250 kilometres, accompanied by two class teachers from the school and four youth workers. They secured the parents' consent through the State Department of Education and the parents were well informed about what was going on. The initiative was designed to last for two days so the students themselves would experience real life as a 'prisoner'. They would feel the difficulties and terrible life of the prisoner – without any freedom and the experience of an extremely dull life.

The result of this first initiative was felt to be very fruitful. Firdaus judged that the majority of the participating problematic students managed to get a great lesson from the prison experience and made significant changes in their behaviour. Firdaus frequently received good feedback from the teachers about the students' behaviour changes when they returned from the programme. He also received spontaneous reactions from the students when they were in the prison cells. The students cried and swore that they would not repeat the same mistakes. They really hated to be put into the cells, even only for one night. In other situations, Firdaus accidentally met some of the ex-participants in the mosques. They had started to become committed Muslims by performing congregational prayer regularly in the mosque.

Following the success of the first initiative, Firdaus decided to plan a second initiative with a new group of school students. Firdaus gave the following account:

Our initiative suddenly became known to a prominent educational figure who was an academic in one of Malaysia's top universities. He was also one of the leaders of one of the most influential associations, namely The National Association of Parents and Teachers. He spontaneously criticised our initiative. His reason was that our initiative involved punishing those problematic students. A school student should not be sent to prison, even it was only for two days and a night. He suggested that other alternatives should replace this initiative. Quite possibly he was strictly interpreting Section 96 (2) of the Child Act (2001), which states that: 'A child aged 14 years or above shall not be ordered to be imprisoned if he can be suitably dealt with in any other way, whether by probation, or fine, or being sent to a place of detention or an approved school, or a Henry Gurney School, or otherwise.' At the same, he did not try to seek clarification from us directly, but instead he criticised us publicly in the mainstream media. We did not have any chance to defend our initiative.

We felt this was an unfair criticism. At that stage, since our intention was to educate the students, we organised the programme for two days and one night only. It was just to expose the students to the real conditions in prison. If our intention was to punish them, we would have definitely organised it for more than two days. But we faced a dilemma about whether to proceed with our second initiative or not. On the one hand, we were afraid that we would receive constant criticism from those who misunderstood the real purpose and context of our initiative, and as a result this would have a negative impact on ABIM. On the other hand, we identified that this was amongst the best intervention initiatives that we had ever had to bring those students back to the right path.

After we had had a discussion among the youth workers involved, making a balanced and fair contemplation on the matter, we firmly resolved to proceed with this initiative quietly, without any media coverage, in the belief that it would bring more positive impacts to the students personally than negative impacts. Despite that, we really regretted, and again it was a dilemma for us, that we could not share this good initiative with the community at large and other NGOs, so that others could use the same kind of initiative when dealing with disciplinary problems in schools. We were more than happy to stress the point that this initiative was deliberately designed to educate through experiential learning (because 'seeing is believing') and not to punish the young people.

Maintaining the rules: a dilemma about a homeless person in Spain

Introduction

This case is set in Spain and was given by a social worker employed in a shelter for homeless people. Most large towns and cities have homeless shelters, which tend to be run through the local public social services system or by NGOs or private organisations. They may be staffed by social workers or other types of staff. They generally have quite strict rules regarding opening and closing times and use of drugs or alcohol.

The case

José (42 years old) is a user of a shelter for homeless people in Burgos, Spain. This public facility is open the whole week, providing night shelter and a space for the development of a social intervention programme. The rules governing the operation of the service include the obligation to stay sober and not to be under the influence of drugs, as well as to respect the time limit to access it, namely that there is no entry after 23.00 hours.

José has been using the shelter for two months and living on the streets for more than 10 years. One night he came to the shelter after the time limit and with clear evidence of alcohol consumption; this happened in winter, during one of the coldest nights of the year. He was quite upset; he claimed his right to spend the night in the shelter and threatened to go away and not come back any more if the staff did not allow him to come in.

This was the first time that this happened in the two months that José had been involved in this social integration programme. The assessment of the progress he has made to date is highly positive.

The other people involved in the programme heard all the noise made by José when he found the door closed. Some of them asked the social worker, who at that moment was in charge of the service, not to leave José in the street, since he might suffer hypothermia. Others said that rules were compulsory for all and that there should be no preferential treatment.

Case 7.6

Balancing a girl's need with a mother's decision: a dilemma for a youth worker in Finland

Introduction

This case is written by a third-year community educator student who was studying the degree programme in Civic Activities and Youth Work in Finland. The student was undertaking her fieldwork practice placement in a 'youth house' in a city in the southern part of Finland. A youth house is a place where young people can spend time with adults and with each other. There are no fees required to attend youth houses, and youth workers encourage young people's involvement in making decisions about the activities offered, decoration of the houses, and so on. The goal is to help young people to participate in decision-making. Having youth houses is the most important part of basic youth work in Finland. There are youth houses in most areas, providing programmes of informal and leisure activities for young people. The youth houses are generally funded by the local government or NGOs.

The case

I did my first work placement in an open access youth house. The target group was girls only, ranging in age from 6–16 years old. The idea of the house is to provide a space and a time for girls to be themselves and to do activities that are enjoyable and educational. The house is open on Tuesdays and Thursdays from 15.00 to 20.00 hours.

The aim of the work is to provide and support different kinds of social activities for and with the girls through play and by using art, handicrafts and so on. My main job was to be with the girls, talk with them, motivate and support them to find new things to do and have fun. In addition to every Tuesday and Thursday when the house was open, I also worked in different clubs as an instructor. Clubs and groups are one activity in the house. Another activity is the 'Big Sister Programme'. Young girls can have 'big sisters' – young women over 18 years old, who take part in a big sister course where they gain information about being a big sister: a role model and an older friend. 'Sister pairs' first meet and get to know each other in the house. Later they meet when and where they want – once, twice or many times per month, depending on the needs of the 'little sister'.

The kinds of girls who attend regularly tend to be those who do not have very wide social networks – who may lack friends or have few hobbies. Some girls also have troubled family lives or experience problems at school. The values underpinning the work with the girls are based on gender sensitive ways of working. This means that every girl must be supported to find her own ways to build her identity and increase her self-esteem. There is no exact model for being a girl or a boy. People's individual features are valued in themselves.

There was this one girl, aged 13 years, who came to the house almost every time when we were open. She was categorised as having learning disabilities. One of the principles in operation at the house was that workers should not be influenced by possible diagnoses or case descriptions made by social workers. However, spending time with the girl I became aware of the fact that she had a rough time with her family, especially her mother. Her mother sounded to be extremely stressed. She had two jobs at the same time and she could not always take care of the three children in the family. The girl was also bullied at school. We, the staff, could tell that the house and the workers meant a lot to her. The mother and the girl fought a lot and sometimes as a punishment the mother banned her daughter from attending the youth house.

This was a hard situation for us workers. Whenever a new girl arrived at the house, she was allowed to look around and stay there for that day. After that we would give her a paper to take home and get approval from her parents to attend the house. Being in good contact with parents was part of our working methods. With this girl it was really challenging from time to time. The mother did not communicate with the house. For example, she was invited by letter together with other parents to visit the house, but she never came. This could also be a reason why the mother banned her daughter. She had a lack of knowledge about the house because she never visited the place.

It felt so unfair for the girl not to be able attend the house, especially since she really appreciated her time there. It was a difficult ethical issue for us as workers to decide whether we should still let the girl come to the house, in spite of the mother's decision to ban her (which we thought was unreasonable).

Using cases and commentaries in teaching and learning

In this second part of the chapter, we will offer some ideas about how cases can be used in teaching and further study, including some short guidelines for writing cases and commentaries. There is a substantial amount of literature on teaching practical ethics in professional contexts, some of which is listed at the end of this chapter. The following exercises offer just a few ideas based around the types of cases and commentaries in this book. The exercises generally assume a group learning situation, but many can be used by individual readers.

Exercise I: Participants analyse a case and reflect on the commentaries

There are many different ways of analysing a case, and most textbooks offer suggestions. For examples of two systematic models for ethical analysis and decision-making drawn from experience in Belgium and Germany, see Goovaerts (2003) and Windheuser (2003). Other approaches outlined by North American and Australian authors include the use of the ethical principles screen (Harrington and Dolgoff 2008) and an inclusive approach (McAuliffe and Chenoweth 2007). Our approach here is more exploratory and less geared towards a decision or solution to an ethical problem.

1 Give out a case from Chapters 2 to 6, without the commentaries.

2 Ask participants individually, or in groups, to analyse the case. The following general questions could be used:

Short set of questions

- What do you think are the main political, legal, cultural or religious factors that need to be borne in mind when examining this case?
- What do you think are the main ethical issues involved in this case?
- If you could ask the author of the case three questions, what would these be?
- If the social worker (or another key person in this case) asked you for advice about what should happen or what should have

happened, what would you say and what ethical arguments would you use to justify your advice?

Longer set of questions

- What is your initial reaction to this case, including any feelings you may have about it?
- In your opinion, what are the ethical issues involved in this case?
- How are the ethical issues linked to any relevant political, legal, cultural or religious factors?
- Would this case present an ethical challenge or dilemma for you if you were the social worker (or another key person) in the case?
- What further information would you need before deciding what should be done in this case?
- On the basis of the information you have here, how would you act in this case if you were the social worker (or another key person) in the case?
- What reasons would you give for deciding to act in this way?
- What kinds of new ethical problems might arise as a result of your decision?
- Do you have any further comments you want to make?

3 Ask participants to reflect on how easy it is to give advice to someone working in a different country, or in a context with which they are not familiar.

4 If they are working in a group, ask participants to reflect on what differences in perspectives they have, and why.

5 Ask participants to consider specific questions relevant to the case, using questions given at the end of the second commentary, or questions devised by the teacher/facilitator.

6 Ask participants to read the two commentaries and consider all or some of the following questions:

- What are the key ethical issues identified by the commentaries?
- How do they differ from each other, and in what ways are the commentaries different from and similar to your own analysis? Why do you think this is?
- Do the commentators use or refer to any ethical theories or approaches, or ethical principles or concepts, either implicitly or explicitly?
- In your opinion, what are the three most useful and interesting points made by the commentators?

- Are there any points made by the commentators with which you disagree, or which you do not understand?
- How has your understanding of this case, and the ethical issues raised by it, developed or changed as a result of reading the commentaries and/or discussing it with other participants?
- What are the key messages raised by this case for service users, practitioners, managers, policy-makers or other stakeholders?
- If you had the power to change the conditions for the service user(s) in this case, what would you do?

Exercise II: Participants analyse a case and write their own commentary

1 Give out a case, or ask participants to choose a case. This may be taken from Chapters 2 to 6 (without the commentaries), or from Chapter 7, or it may be a case written by one of the participants or a teacher.

2 Ask participants individually or in groups to analyse the case as described in Exercise I.2.

3 Ask participants to do one of the following tasks:

- Write their own commentary on the case (without reading the published commentaries, if the case is from Chapters 2 to 6).
- Read the case with its two commentaries (if the case is from Chapters 2 to 6) and then write their own commentary, taking account of the case *and* the two published commentaries.

4 Give participants the following guidelines for writing a commentary:

- *Audience.* Think about who the readers of your commentary might be. Are the readers likely to be students, teachers, professional practitioners, service users or others? What country are they from, what language do they speak and what knowledge do you think they will have of any theories, social welfare systems and practices to which you may refer? Adjust your language so that what you are saying and how you say it is comprehensible to your audience.
- *Ethical issues.* Highlight what you think are the key ethical issues in the case – how can they be understood? You can discuss the case in relation to different ethical theories, if you wish.
- *Structure.* Use a logical structure – if you think headings would help the reader, then use headings to structure your commentary.

- *Reflection on context.* If you are from a different country than the country of the case, or a different area of work, you might like to reflect on similar issues in your own country or area of work – to what extent are these universal/general questions in a particular context?
- *Stick to the information given.* Be careful only to relate to information that is given in the case. You may wish to speculate about what might have happened or what might have caused a situation, but make it clear that you are speculating. Do not make assumptions about facts in the specific case or country.
- *Think about how critical or judgemental you should be.* Think about how the author of the case, or other people who feature in the case, might respond to your comments. Whilst it is important that you write an honest commentary, from your own perspective, be careful how you phrase any judgements or criticisms in order to minimise unnecessary upset.
- *Ending.* End the commentary with a conclusion, which could be your own position statement ('My opinion about this particular case is . . .' or 'At the heart of this problem lies . . .') or a proposed solution to the problem or another suitable ending to the commentary.
- *Length.* The commentary could be of 500–1000 words in length.

Exercise III: Participants research issues raised by a case and commentaries

1   Ask participants to collect further background material relevant to a particular case.

- If it is set in a different country, what can they discover about social work in that country? If it is set in their home country, what can be found out about the specialist area of practice or policy featured in the case?
- If reference is made to specific laws, policies or guidelines, can more details be found out about these in a language participants can understand?
- If the case raises issues about political conflict, religious or cultural norms, what further relevant information can be obtained about these matters?
- If commentators refer to specific theories or literature, can further reading be undertaken to find out more?

2 How does this background material help us understand the issues raised by the case?

Exercise IV: Using cases as a basis for dialogue, discussion or debate

The teaching of ethics lends itself to the use of dialogical and debating methods. Philippart (2003) offers a useful account of how to facilitate a Socratic dialogue, based on a Dutch model, as a way of getting participants to generate their own examples (which are in effect cases) and then focusing on one case example to answer a general philosophical question (such as, 'What is justice?'). Dialogical methods can also be used to explore a case given out in advance (rather than generated by participants during the dialogue) as follows:

1 Select a case and ask all participants to read it.

2 Choose one of the following exercises:

- Ask participants to form small groups to discuss the issues raised by the case and what should be done in cases like this.
- Facilitate a large group dialogue on the case, encouraging participants to engage with each other rather than the facilitator, with the role of the facilitator being to ensure the dialogue moves on and engages as many participants as possible.

     i The dialogue process could focus on the group collectively undertaking an analysis of the case.
     ii Using the case as a starting point, the dialogue could focus on an abstract question relevant to the case (e.g., in relation to Case 3.3 about the boy with Duchenne Muscular Dystrophy in Vietnam, the question for discussion could be: 'When is it right to withhold information from a family about their child's medical condition?'). Or the focus of the dialogue could be to analyse a case with the purpose of finding the basic values in the case.
     iii Alternatively, two cases could be selected, which are both relevant to the question posed, and the discussion could compare and contrast the circumstances in each case. For example, Case 4.2 about the young man waiting for a transplant in the UK could be compared with Case 3.3 about the sick boy in Vietnam.

- If there are polarised views expressed in the case, or in the two commentaries, or if there could be at least two alternative responses to the case (this action was right/wrong; the social worker should have done X/Y), ask two participants to take alternative positions and make the arguments as strongly as they can for each position. For example, in Case 4.2, one set of arguments could be developed as to why it was right to withhold information from the young man and his family about the fact that he had been removed from the transplant list; and another set of arguments could be developed as to why this action was morally wrong. The rest of the participants can then be invited to ask the questions of the two debaters, and engage in debate themselves in relation to the two positions. Such a 'debate' will be somewhat artificial. However, this exercise serves to focus attention on the nature of ethical arguments; the ways in which apparently polarised positions may be less polarised than we think; and how there may be other positions available in addition to the two presented.

Exercise V: Using cases as a basis for drama or role play

A case can be used as the subject of a dramatic performance or role play in a class or a team meeting. This can help participants explore how a situation may be experienced from the perspective of a particular character, and may give the opportunity to rehearse how alternative responses to a situation could be acted out. Langen (2003) gives some examples of the use of drama in exploring ethical theory with social work students in Switzerland based on *Themenzentriertes Theater*. This approach could be adapted to explore themes (such as 'respect', or 'dignity') based on cases. Doing a role play based on a case is another possibility, as follows:

1   Choose a case. For illustrative purposes, let us assume that Case 4.2 about the young man waiting for an organ transplant in a hospital has been chosen.

2   Participants could be asked to take on the roles of the young man, his parents, the social worker, the hospital consultant, two nurses and any other characters that might be involved.

3   A short scenario based on the written case could be acted out. For example, the scenario might be a team meeting of the professionals

involved in the case when the young man's deteriorating condition is discussed; the decision is made to take him off the waiting list for a transplant and not to inform him or his family. A second scenario could be developed involving the young man and his family, in which the consultant talks to the young man and his family about his worsening condition but does not actually tell them that his name has been taken off the list. The social worker might then stay with the family to discuss issues further with them.

4   Feedback could then be taken from the 'actors' in the role play, and comments made by other participants observing the action. The observers could be asked to look out for words, actions and movements that they think might signify empathy, respect, lack of respect or parentalism, for example. Suggestions might be made for alternative ways in which the consultant and social worker could talk with the family, including informing them about the decision, and the people playing these roles could act out the suggestions. One of the observers might then take over the role of the social worker to try out a different approach, which could then be evaluated by the 'actors' involved and the observers.

5   Care should be taken to 'debrief' the actors afterwards (asking how it felt for them in the role). Facilitators or teachers need to be aware of emotions that can be stirred up by role play and be prepared to handle these. In an emotive case like this, it is highly likely that it may be upsetting for some participants.

Exercise VI: Participants write their own cases

Participants can be asked to write their own cases for use in class, web-based discussion, group supervisions or team discussions (see Banks and Nyboe 2003). The following guidance may be helpful:

1   *What is a case?* A case can be regarded as a short description of a situation, an event or a piece of work. We are looking for a case that gives an account of a real situation, describing the important features. The case may describe everyday events and actions that a social worker, other professional, student, carer or service user encounters in practice; or it may be a description of a situation that is constructed as problematic – involving a difficult decision, a dilemma, or a situation where 'mistakes' have been made.

2 *Selection of relevant material.* Cases are always 'constructed', that is, the writer decides what features of the situation are relevant and how to put them into words. A case can be based on a situation in which you yourself played a role or on a story told to you by somebody else. A case might be based on an interview.

3 *The art of writing a case.* Writing a good case is an art – to ensure clarity, interest and sufficient (but not too much) information. The following checklist of points to bear in mind might be helpful:

- Does the case give a clear description of the situation?
- Does the case give the reader sufficient information to make it interesting and comprehensible, but not so many details that the reader may be confused?
- Does the case have a clear storyline (a 'main thread')?
- Does the case have the potential to generate discussion (does it raise challenging ethical questions, is it controversial, open ended)?

4 *Background information.* It is often helpful if the writer of a case can also preface it with a short introduction about the national, social, cultural and political context in which the case takes place and, if relevant, a note on any legal or 'local' issues.

5 *Anonymity.* A case should always be carefully anonymised, with names of people, organisations and places changed and any identifying features removed or changed, in order to protect the identity of the people and organisations involved. Sometimes the authors of cases may also wish to remain anonymous, to ensure that their identities do not reveal the identities of other people or organisations, especially if the content of the case is personally or politically sensitive.

Exercise VII: Using cases in web-based learning

Many of these exercises could be adapted for web-based, distance learning and blended learning contexts. Participants could write commentaries on each others' cases, post them on the worldwide web and engage in further dialogue with each other – making short comments and asking questions. Bozalek (2010) offers a useful outline of the use of blended learning in teaching social work ethics in South Africa.

Exercise VIII: Using a case as a basis for a written assignment

A case, or a case and the accompanying commentaries, could be used as a basis for a written assignment. Students could be asked to write their own analysis of the case (see Exercise I.2) or their own commentary (see Exercise II.4). Pettersson (2003: 139) gives an example of using a case in a written examination of a social work course in Sweden.

References

Note: The complete book, Banks, S. and Nøhr, K. (2003) *Teaching Practical Ethics for the Social Professions*, Copenhagen: FESET, is freely available for downloading at www.feset.org/en/hom-groups/esep.html e/activities/thematic

Banks, S. and Nyboe, N.-E. (2003) 'Writing and using cases', in S. Banks and K. Nøhr (eds) *Teaching Practical Ethics for the Social Professions*, Copenhagen: FESET.

Bozalek, V. (2010) 'Moral dilemmas in a South African blended learning ethics course ', in D. Zaviršek, B. Rommelspacher and S. Staub-Bernasconi (eds) *Ethical Dilemmas in Social Work: International Perspective*, Ljubljana: Faculty of Social Work, University of Ljubljana.

Fook, J. and Askeland, G. (2006) 'The "critical" in critical reflection', in S. White, J. Fook and F. Gardner (eds) *Critical Reflection in Health and Social Care*, Maidenhead: Open University Press.

Goovaerts, H. (2003) 'Working with a staged plan', in S. Banks and K. Nøhr (eds) *Teaching Practical Ethics for the Social Professions*, Copenhagen: FESET.

Harrington, D. and Dolgoff, R. (2008) 'Hierarchies of ethical principles for ethical decision making in social work', *Ethics and Social Welfare* 2(2): 183–196.

Langen, R. (2003) 'Exploring aspects of ethical theory through drama', in S. Banks and K. Nøhr (eds) *Teaching Practical Ethics for the Social Professions*, Copenhagen: FESET.

McAuliffe, D. and Chenoweth, L. (2007) 'Leave no stone unturned: The inclusive model of ethical decision-making', *Ethics and Social Welfare* 2(1): 38–49.

Pettersson, H. (2003) 'Integrating the teaching of ethics into the curriculum', in S. Banks and K. Nøhr (eds) *Teaching Practical Ethics for the Social Professions*, Copenhagen: FESET.

Philippart, F. (2003) 'Using Socratic dialogue', in S. Banks and K. Nøhr (eds) *Teaching Practical Ethics for the Social Professions*, Copenhagen: FESET.

Schön, D. (1991) *The Reflective Practitioner: How Professionals Think in Action*, Aldershot: Avebury/Ashgate.

Taylor, C. (2006) 'Practising reflexivity: narrative, reflection and the moral order', in S. White, J. Fook and F. Gardner (eds) *Critical Reflection in Health and Social Care*, Maidenhead: Open University Press.

Windheuser, J. (2003) 'An ethical decision-making model', in S. Banks and K. Nøhr (eds) *Teaching Practical Ethics for the Social Professions*, Copenhagen: FESET.

Index